Welcome Home

ONE-POT
FAVORITES

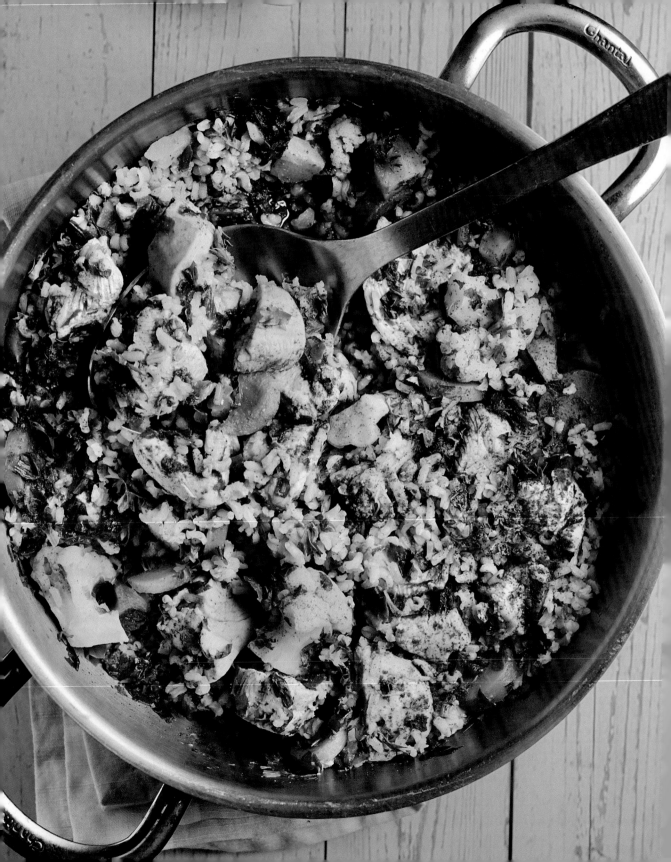

Welcome Home
ONE-POT FAVORITES

SHEET PAN, SKILLET, INSTANT POT & DUTCH OVEN MEALS

Hope Comerford

Photos by Bonnie Matthews

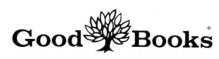

Good Books

New York, New York

Copyright © 2025 by Good Books
Photos by Bonnie Matthews

Good Books books may be purchased in bulk at special discounts for sales
promotion, corporate gifts, fund-raising, or educational purposes. Special
editions can also be created to specifications. For details, contact the Special Sales
Department, Good Books, 307 West 36th Street, 11th Floor, New York, NY 10018
or info@skyhorsepublishing.com.

Good Books is an imprint of Skyhorse Publishing, Inc.®, a Delaware corporation.

Visit our website at www.goodbooks.com.

10 9 8 7 6 5 4 3 2 1

Library of Congress Cataloging-in-Publication Data is available on file.

Cover design by Kai Texel
Cover photo by Bonnie Matthews

Print ISBN: 978-1-68099-962-4
Ebook ISBN: 978-1-68099-979-2

Printed in China

Table of Contents

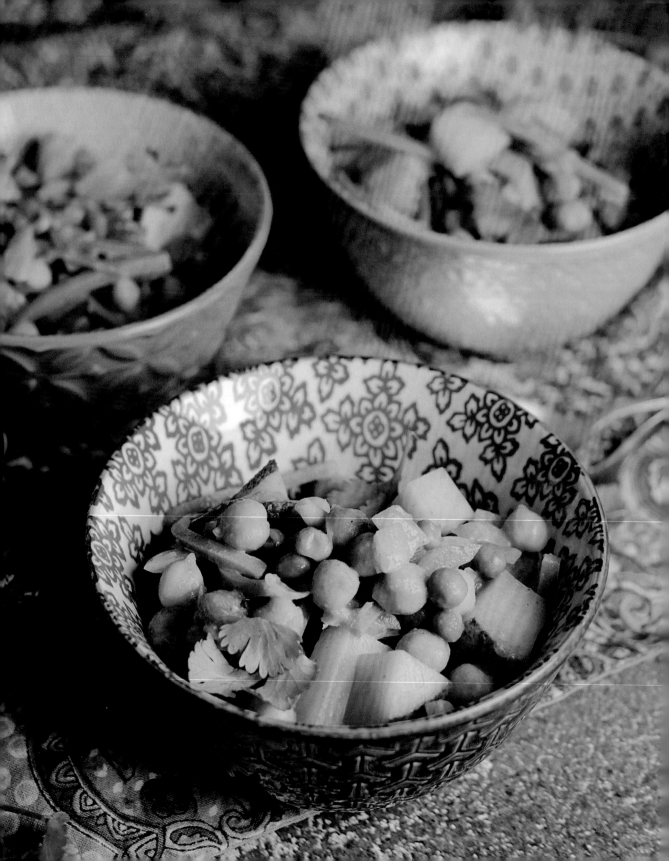

About Welcome Home One-Pot Favorites!

We know your time is precious. You don't have time to clean a pile of dishes just to get a home-cooked meal on the table. You also don't have time to scour the grocery store, searching for complicated ingredients, only to come home and prepare a complicated recipe. *Welcome Home One-Pot Favorites* will provide you with homemade, tasty meal to serve your family, while still having time to enjoy their company.

Within these pages, you'll find 127 recipes for the slow-cooker, Instant Pot, stovetop, oven, Dutch oven, grill, and even recipes that require no cooking! All the recipes are easy to follow and quick to prepare. You do not need to be an experienced cook to follow these tried-and-true recipes.

As you begin journeying through this book, I always suggest reading it from cover to cover. I can't tell you the good recipes I've passed on in the past by not following this advice. Don't become overwhelmed. Bookmark or dog-ear the pages of the recipes that you think your family would enjoy the most, can be made with ingredients you have around the house, or fit with their dietary needs. Then, when you've looked at everything, go back to those marked pages and narrow it down. Make yourself a grocery list and grab what you don't already have. Voilà! You're ready to get cooking!

Breakfasts

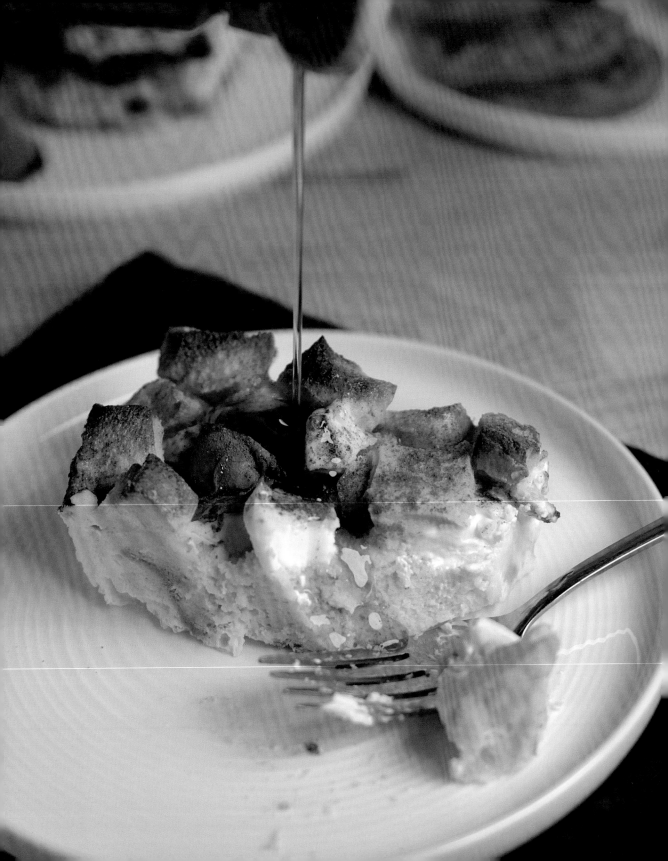

French Toast Casserole

OVEN

Stacy Stoltzfus, Grantham, PA
Kaye Taylor, Florissant, MO

Makes 12 servings

Prep. Time: 10–15 minutes ✿ *Chilling Time: Overnight* ✿ *Baking Time: 45 minutes*

10 slices bread, cubed, *divided*

2 (8-oz.) pkg. cream cheese

12 eggs, beaten well

2 cups milk

Cinnamon, *optional*

1. Place half of the bread cubes in a greased 9 × 13-inch pan.

2. Cube the cream cheese and scatter on top of the bread.

3. Put the rest of the bread cubes on top.

4. In a large bowl, use an electric mixer to beat the eggs and milk. Pour the mixture over the top of the bread and cream cheese.

5. Sprinkle the top with cinnamon, if you wish.

6. Refrigerate overnight. In the morning, bake at 375°F for 45 minutes. Cut into squares or dish out with a spoon.

Tip:

You can add fruit scattered with the cream cheese cubes: berries, diced apples, peaches, etc.

Serving suggestion:

Serve hot with syrup. (Fruit syrups are especially good.)

SLOW
COOKER

Blueberry Fancy

Leticia A. Zehr, Lowville, NY

Makes 12 servings

Prep. Time: 10–15 minutes ⚜ *Cooking Time: 3–4 hours* ⚜ *Ideal slow-cooker size: 5-qt.*

I loaf Italian bread, cubed, *divided*
I pt. blueberries, *divided*
8 oz. cream cheese, cubed, *divided*
6 eggs
1½ cups milk
I tsp. vanilla extract

1. Spray the crock with nonstick spray.

2. Place half the bread cubes in the slow cooker.

3. Drop half the blueberries over top the bread.

4. Sprinkle half the cream cheese cubes over the blueberries.

5. Repeat all 3 layers.

6. In a mixing bowl, whisk together the eggs, milk, and vanilla. Pour over all ingredients in the slow cooker.

7. Cover and cook on Low for 3–4 hours, until the dish is custardy and set.

8. Serve with maple syrup or blueberry sauce.

Baked Oatmeal

Lena Sheaffer, Port Matilda, PA
Susie Nissley, Millersburg, OH
Esther Nafziger, Bluffton, OH
Katie Stoltzfus, Leola, PA
Martha Hershey, Ronks, PA
Annabelle Unternahrer, Shipshewana, IN

Makes 4–6 servings

Prep. Time: 10 minutes ❧ *Baking Time: 30 minutes*

½ cup oil

1 cup honey or brown sugar

2 eggs

3 cups rolled or quick oats, uncooked

2 tsp. baking powder

1 cup milk

½ tsp. cinnamon or nutmeg, *optional*

1 cup chopped nuts, raisins, apples, or other fruit

1. Combine oil, honey or brown sugar, and eggs in a large mixing bowl.

2. Add dry oats, baking powder, and milk. Add spice if using. Mix well.

3. Add nuts and/or fruit. Mix well.

4. Pour into a greased 8-inch-square baking pan.

5. Bake at 350°F for 30 minutes.

6. Serve hot, cold, or at room temperature with milk.

Variations:

Add any or all of these: ½ cup dried cherries, ½ cup dried cranberries, ½ cup cut-up apricots.

Country Brunch

Esther J. Mast, Lancaster, PA
Barbara Yoder, Christiana, PA
Ruth Ann Gingrich, New Holland, PA
Lafaye Musser, Denver, PA

Makes 12–15 servings

Prep. Time: 30 minutes ⚹ Chilling Time: 8 hours, or overnight
Baking Time: 45–60 minutes ⚹ Standing Time: 10–15 minutes

16 slices firm white bread

1⅔–2 lb. (2½ cups) cubed ham or browned sausage, drained

1 lb. (3 cups) shredded cheddar cheese

1 lb. (3 cups) shredded mozzarella cheese

8 eggs, beaten

3½ cups milk

½ tsp. mustard powder

¼ tsp. onion powder

½ tsp. seasoning salt

1 Tbsp. parsley

Topping:

3 cups uncrushed cornflakes

8 Tbsp. (1 stick) butter, melted

1. Trim crusts from bread and cut slices in half.

2. Grease a 10 × 15-inch baking dish.

3. Layer ingredients in this order: cover bottom of pan with half the bread, top with half the ham, then half the cheddar cheese, and then half the mozzarella cheese.

4. Repeat layers once more.

5. In large mixing bowl, combine eggs, milk, mustard, onion powder, seasoning salt, and parsley. Mix well and pour over layers.

6. Cover and refrigerate for 8 hours, or overnight.

7. Remove from refrigerator 30 minutes before baking.

8. Combine cornflakes and butter and sprinkle over casserole.

9. Cover loosely with foil to prevent over-browning. Bake at 375°F for 45 minutes.

10. Remove from oven and let stand 10–15 minutes before cutting into squares.

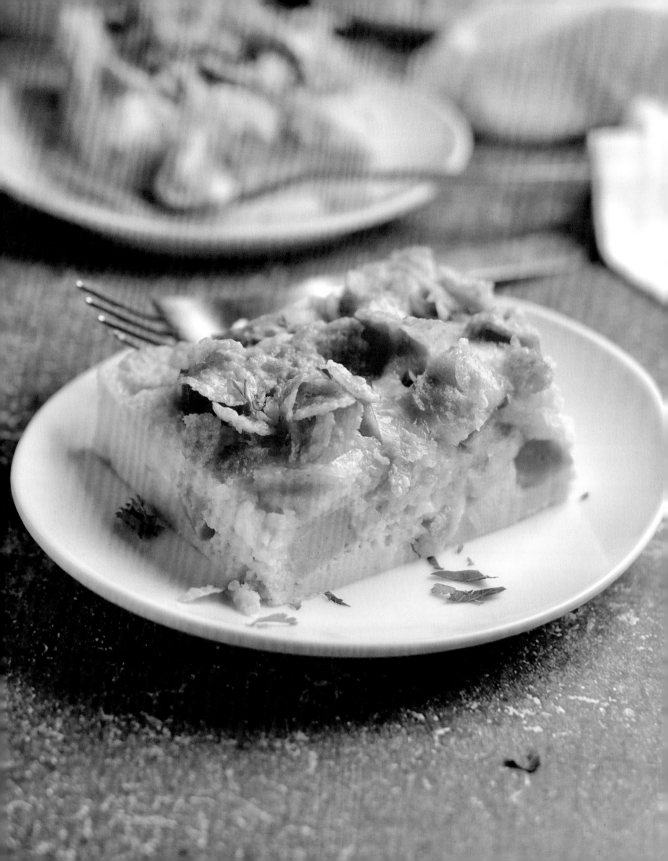

Biscuits and Gravy the Instant Pot Way

Hope Comerford, Clinton Township, MI

Makes 4 servings

Prep. Time: 5 minutes   ⚬   Cooking Time: 16–20 minutes

Gravy:

I Tbsp. butter

8 oz. bulk breakfast sausage

3 Tbsp. flour

½ tsp. garlic powder

¼ tsp. sea salt

¼ tsp. black pepper

1½ cups milk

Biscuits:

¾ cup baking mix

⅓ cup milk

¼ tsp. black pepper

¼ tsp. sea salt

1. Set the Instant Pot to the Sauté setting and place the butter in the inner pot to melt.

2. Add in the breakfast sausage and sauté until browned, about 8 minutes.

3. Stir in the flour, garlic powder, sea salt, and pepper.

4. Whisk in the milk, and bring to a simmer, stirring occasionally.

5. Press Cancel on the Instant Pot.

6. In a bowl, mix the biscuit ingredients.

7. Place dollops of the biscuit mixture over the gravy.

8. Secure the lid and set the vent to sealing.

9. Manually set the cook time for 4 minutes.

10. When cook time is up, let the pressure release naturally for 5 minutes, then manually release the remaining pressure.

11. Serve and enjoy!

Breakfast Sausage Ring

Joanne E. Martin, Stevens, PA

Makes 8 servings

Prep. Time: 15 minutes ❧ *Baking Time: 40–45 minutes* ❧ *Standing Time: 10 minutes*

2 lb. bulk pork sausage
2 eggs, beaten
1½ cups fine dry breadcrumbs
¼ cup chopped parsley, *optional*
Salt and pepper to taste, *optional*

1. Lightly grease a 9-inch oven-safe ring mold.

2. In a large mixing bowl, mix all ingredients well. Then pack into the mold.

3. Bake at 350°F for 20 minutes.

4. Remove from the oven and pour off any accumulated fat. Return to oven to bake for 20 minutes more.

5. Remove from the oven and allow to stand for 10 minutes. Turn onto a platter.

Serving suggestion:
Fill the center of the Sausage Ring with scrambled eggs before serving.

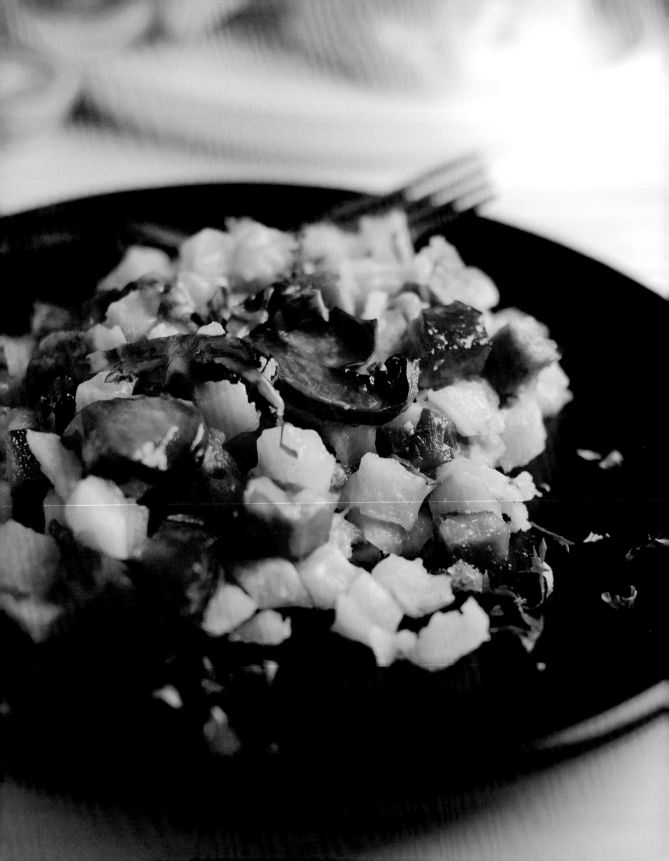

Ham and Mushroom Hashbrowns

SLOW COOKER

Evelyn Page, Riverton, WY
Anna Stoltzfus, Honey Brook, PA

Makes: 6–8 servings

Prep. Time: 15 minutes & Cooking Time: 6–8 hours & Ideal slow-cooker size: 5-qt.

28-oz. pkg. frozen hash brown potatoes

2½ cups cubed cooked ham

2-oz. jar pimentos, drained and chopped

4-oz. can mushrooms, or ¼ lb. sliced fresh mushrooms

10¾-oz. can cheddar cheese soup

¾ cup half-and-half

Dash pepper

Salt to taste

1. Combine potatoes, ham, pimentos, and mushrooms in slow cooker.

2. Combine soup, half-and-half, and seasonings. Pour over potatoes.

3. Cover. Cook on Low 6–8 hours.

Tip:

If you turn the cooker on when you go to bed, you'll have a wonderfully tasty breakfast in the morning.

OVEN

Mom's Heavenly Quiche

Barbara Forrester Landis, Lititz, PA

Makes 6–8 servings

Prep. Time: 15 minutes 🍂 Baking Time: 40–50 minutes

6 eggs, or equivalent amount
of egg substitute

2 Tbsp. flour

2 cups cottage cheese

1 cup shredded cheddar cheese

4 Tbsp. (½ stick) butter, melted

4-oz. can diced green chiles,
undrained, *optional*

Tips:

• You can use any kind of
flour. I use whole wheat.

• You can use any kind of
cottage cheese. I use low-
fat.

• This is delicious eaten cold
the next day if there's any
left.

• If you have leftover cooked
veggies in your refrigerator,
place them in the bottom of
the pan and cover with egg
mixture as a variation.

1. In a good-sized mixing bowl, beat the eggs or pour in egg substitute.

2. Stir in the flour.

3. When well mixed, stir in the cottage cheese, shredded cheese, and butter, and the diced green chiles, if using.

4. Pour into a greased 10-inch pie plate.

5. Bake for 40–45 minutes, or until set in center. Insert the blade of a knife in the center. If it comes out clean, the quiche is finished. If it doesn't, bake for 5 more minutes. Test again, and continue baking if needed.

6. Let stand 10 minutes before cutting to allow cheeses to firm up.

Crustless Spinach Quiche

SLOW COOKER

Barbara Hoover, Landisville, PA

Makes 8 servings

Prep. Time: 15 minutes ⚬ *Cooking Time: 2–4 hours* ⚬ *Ideal slow-cooker size: 3- or 4-qt.*

2 (10-oz.) pkgs. frozen chopped spinach

2 cups cottage cheese

4 Tbsp. (½ stick) butter, cut into pieces

1½ cups sharp cheese, cubed

3 eggs, beaten

¼ cup flour

1 tsp. salt

1. Grease interior of slow-cooker crock.

2. Thaw spinach completely. Squeeze as dry as you can. Then place in crock.

3. Stir in all other ingredients and combine well.

4. Cover. Cook on Low for 2–4 hours, or until quiche is set. Stick blade of knife into center of quiche. If blade comes out clean, quiche is set. If it doesn't, cover and cook another 15 minutes or so.

5. When cooked, allow to stand for 10–15 minutes so mixture can firm up. Then serve.

Variations:

- Double the recipe if you wish. Cook it in a 5-qt. slow cooker.

- Omit cottage cheese. Add 1 cup milk, 1 tsp. baking powder, and increase flour to 1 cup instead.

- Reserve sharp cheese and sprinkle on top. Allow to melt before serving.

—Barbara Jean Fabel

OVEN

Cheddar-Ham Oven Omelet

Jolene Schrock, Millersburg, OH

Makes 9–12 servings

*Prep. Time: 10 minutes * ❧ * Baking Time: 40–45 minutes * ❧ * Standing Time: 10 minutes*

16 eggs

2 cups milk

8 oz. shredded cheddar cheese

¾ cup cubed fully cooked ham

6 scallions

Chopped sliced mushrooms, *optional*

Chopped green peppers, *optional*

1. In a large bowl, beat the eggs and milk until well blended. Stir in the cheese and ham. Add the scallions and the mushrooms and green peppers, if using.

2. Pour the egg mixture into a greased 9 × 13-inch baking dish.

3. Bake, uncovered, at 350°F for 40–45 minutes, or until a knife inserted near the center comes out clean. Let stand 10 minutes before cutting and serving.

Variation:

Add ½ tsp. salt and ¼ tsp. pepper, if you wish, to Step 1.

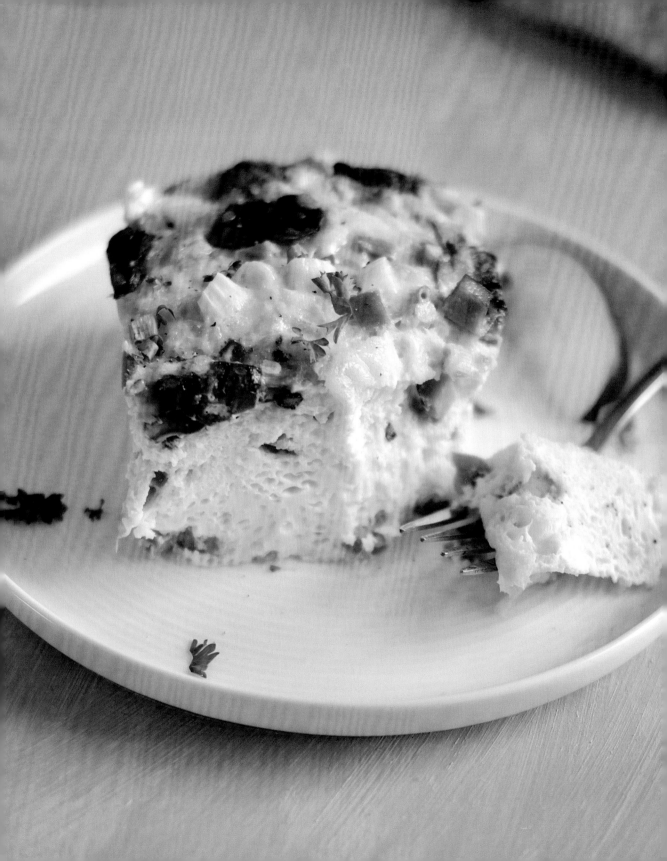

Western Omelet

Mary Louise Martin, Boyd, WI
Jan Mast, Lancaster, PA

Makes: 10 servings

Prep. Time: 15 minutes ❧ *Cooking Time: 4–6 hours* ❧ *Ideal slow-cooker size: 5-qt.*

32-oz. bag frozen hash brown potatoes, *divided*

1 lb. cooked ham, cubed, *divided*

1 medium onion, diced, *divided*

1½ cups shredded cheddar cheese, *divided*

18 eggs

1½ cups milk

1 tsp. salt

1 tsp. pepper

1. Grease interior of slow-cooker crock. Layer ⅓ each of frozen potatoes, ham, onion, and cheese in bottom of slow cooker.

2. Repeat 2 times.

3. Beat together eggs, milk, salt, and pepper in a large mixing bowl. Pour over mixture in slow cooker.

4. Cover. Cook on Low 4–6 hours, or until potatoes are fully cooked and omelet is firm but not dry or overcooked.

Serving suggestion:

This is a great breakfast, served along with orange juice and fresh fruit.

California Egg Bake

Leona M. Slabaugh, Apple Creek, OH

Makes 2 servings

Prep. Time: 10–15 minutes   *Baking Time: 25–30 minutes*

3 eggs

¼ cup sour cream

¼ tsp. salt

1 medium tomato, chopped

1 scallion, sliced

¼ cup shredded cheese

1. In a small bowl, beat eggs, sour cream, and salt.

2. Stir in tomato, scallion, and cheese.

3. Pour into greased 2-cup baking dish.

4. Bake at 350°F for 25–30 minutes, or until a knife inserted in center comes out clean.

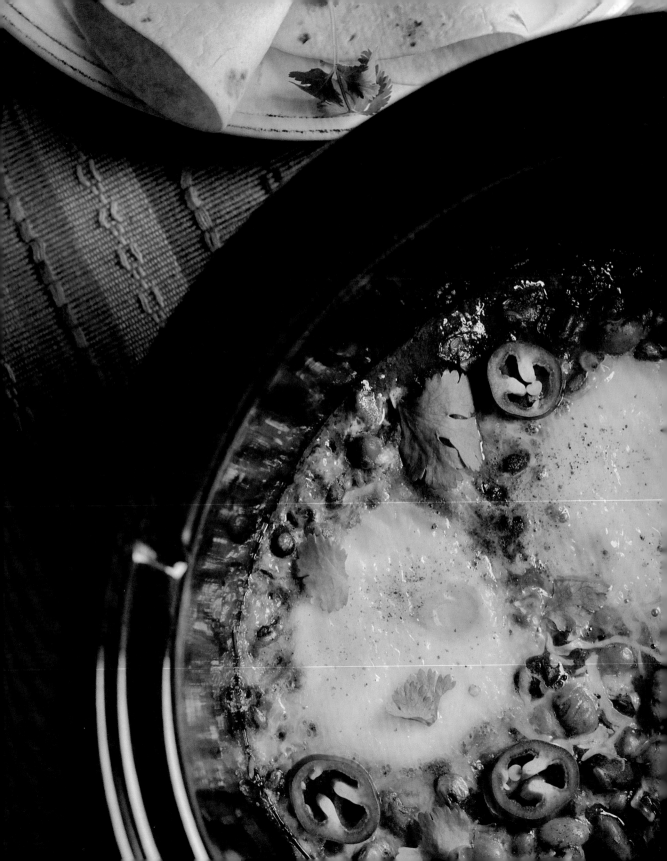

Huevos Rancheros

Pat Bishop, Bedminster, PA

Makes 6 servings

Prep. Time: 25 minutes ⚬ *Cooking Time: 2 hours* ⚬ *Ideal slow-cooker size: 6-qt.*

3 cups gluten-free salsa, room temperature

2 cups cooked beans, drained, room temperature

6 eggs, room temperature

Salt and pepper to taste

⅓ cup reduced-fat grated Mexican-blend cheese, *optional*

1. In a slow cooker, mix the salsa and beans.

2. Cook on High for 1 hour or until steaming.

3. With a spoon, make 6 evenly spaced dents in the salsa mixture; try not to expose the bottom of the crock. Break an egg into each dent.

4. Salt and pepper the eggs. Sprinkle with the cheese, if using.

5. Cover and continue to cook on High until the egg whites are set and the yolks are as firm as you like them, approximately 20–40 minutes.

6. To serve, scoop out an egg with some beans and salsa.

Serving suggestion:
Serve with warm white corn tortillas.

Mexican Breakfast Casserole

Hope Comerford, Clinton Township, MI

Makes 4 servings

Prep. Time: 20 minutes & Cooking Time: 7–8 hours & Ideal slow-cooker size: 3-qt.

8 eggs

1½ cups milk

1 tsp. salt

1 tsp. pepper

¾ cup picante sauce

1 small onion, chopped

½ jalapeño pepper, seeds removed, minced

1 cup frozen corn

2 cups shredded Mexican blend cheese, *divided*

9 (or more) white corn tortillas (5¾-inch recommended)

7 oz. (or so) chorizo, removed from the casing, *divided*

1. Mix the eggs, milk, salt, pepper, picante sauce, onion, jalapeño, corn, and 1 cup shredded Mexican blend cheese.

2. Spray your crock with nonstick spray.

3. Line the bottom of the crock with approximately 3 white corn tortillas.

4. Pour half of the egg mixture over this and then crumble half of the chorizo on top. Repeat this process with another layer of tortillas, egg mixture, and the remaining chorizo.

5. Top with a final layer of tortillas and the remaining cheese on top.

6. Cover and cook on Low for 7–8 hours.

Soups, Stews & Chilies

Chicken

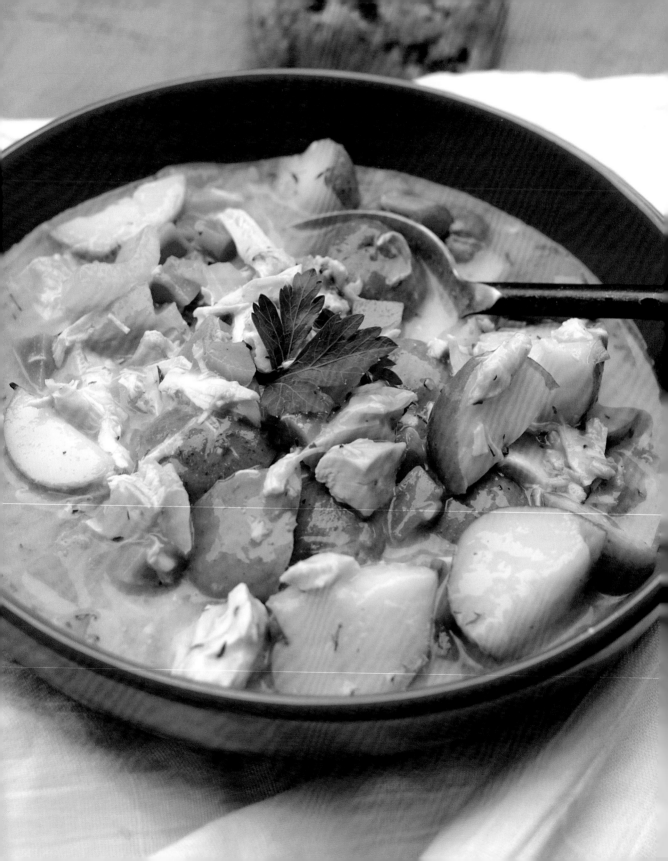

Chicken Stew

Hope Comerford, Clinton Township, MI

Makes 6 servings

Prep. Time: 10 minutes ⚬ *Cooking Time: 20 minutes*

1 Tbsp. olive oil

1 cup chopped onion

3 carrots, chopped

2 celery stalks, chopped

4 cups chicken broth, *divided*

2 lb. boneless, skinless chicken breasts, diced

4–5 red potatoes, chopped

2½ tsp. salt

3 tsp. garlic powder

3 tsp. onion powder

1½ tsp. Italian seasoning

¼ tsp. pepper

2 bay leaves

2 Tbsp. cornstarch

2 Tbsp. cold water

1. Press Sauté on the Instant Pot. Let it get hot. Add the oil.

2. Sauté the onion, carrots, and celery for about 3–5 minutes.

3. Pour in 1 cup of the broth and scrape the bottom of the inner pot to bring up any stuck-on bits. Press Cancel.

4. Add the chicken, red potatoes, salt, garlic powder, onion powder, Italian seasoning, pepper, bay leaves, and remaining 3 cups of broth.

5. Secure the lid and set the vent to sealing. Manually set the cook time for 10 minutes on high pressure.

6. When cook time is up, let the pressure release naturally for 10 minutes, then manually release the remaining pressure. When the pin drops, remove the lid. Press Cancel.

7. Press the Sauté function once again. Mix the cornstarch and cold water, then stir it into the stew. Let it simmer for about 5 minutes, or until it is thickened. Remove the bay leaves before serving.

Tip:

My family loves stew with crusty Italian or French bread with butter on top.

Chicken Noodle Soup

Colleen Heatwole, Burton, MI

Makes 8 servings

Prep. Time: 15 minutes   *Cooking Time: 45–50 minutes*

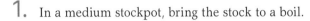

2½ qt. chicken stock
½ cup diced celery
½ cup diced carrots
8-oz. pkg. egg noodles
2 cups cooked, diced chicken
Salt, *optional*

1. In a medium stockpot, bring the stock to a boil.

2. Add the celery and carrots. Simmer for about 7 minutes, or until the vegetables are tender but not overcooked.

3. Add the noodles and chicken. Return the soup to a boil. Continue to cook for another 5–7 minutes, or until the noodles are tender but not mushy.

4. Add salt, if using.

Chunky Chicken Vegetable Soup

Janice Muller, Derwood, MD

Makes 6 servings

Prep. Time: 20 minutes ⚭ *Cooking Time: 2–6 hours* ⚭ *Ideal slow-cooker size: 3½- to 4-qt.*

2½ cups water

8-oz. can tomato sauce

10-oz. pkg. frozen mixed vegetables, partially thawed

1½ tsp. Italian seasoning

1 pkg. dry chicken noodle soup mix

2 cups chopped cooked chicken or turkey

1. In a slow cooker, combine all the ingredients.

2. Cook on Low for 2–6 hours, depending upon how crunchy you like your vegetables.

Tip:

This is a great soup to make with some leftover turkey from Thanksgiving dinner.

Chicken Tortellini Soup

Mary Seielstad, Sparks, NV

Makes 4–6 servings

Prep. Time: 10–15 minutes 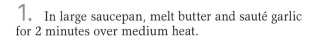 *Cooking Time: 25 minutes*

1 Tbsp. butter or margarine
4 cloves garlic, minced
5 cups chicken broth
9-oz. pkg. frozen cheese tortellini
1½ cups diced cooked chicken
14-oz. can stewed tomatoes
10-oz. pkg. frozen spinach
½ tsp. pepper
1 tsp. dried basil
¼ cup grated Parmesan cheese

1. In large saucepan, melt butter and sauté garlic for 2 minutes over medium heat.

2. Stir in broth and tortellini and bring to a boil. Cover, reduce heat, and simmer 5 minutes.

3. Add cooked chicken, tomatoes, frozen spinach, pepper, and basil and simmer 10–15 minutes. Stir every 3 minutes or so, breaking up frozen spinach and blending it into the soup.

4. Serve when soup is heated through, along with Parmesan cheese to spoon over individual servings.

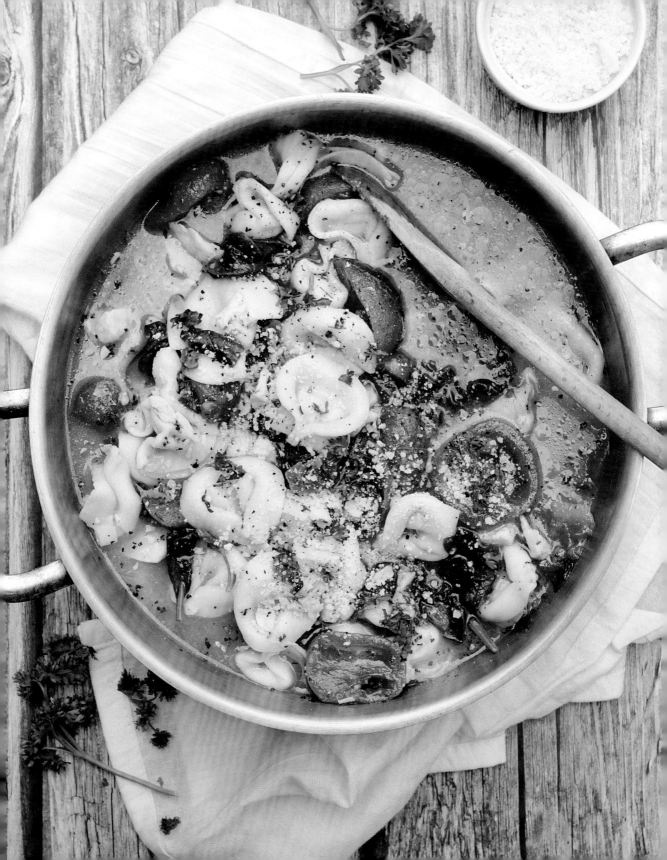

Quick Taco Chicken Soup

Karen Waggoner, Joplin, MO

Makes 4–6 servings

Prep. Time: 5 minutes ❧ *Cooking Time: 1 hour* ❧ *Ideal slow-cooker size: 4-qt.*

12-oz. can cooked chicken, undrained

14-oz. can chicken broth

16-oz. jar mild thick-and-chunky salsa

15-oz. can ranch-style beans

15-oz. can whole-kernel corn

1. In a slow cooker, combine all the ingredients.

2. Cover and cook on High for 1 hour. Keep warm on Low until ready to serve.

Black Bean Soup with Chicken and Salsa

Hope Comerford, Clinton Township, MI

Makes 4–6 servings

Prep. Time: 10 minutes ⚬ Cooking Time: 6–8 hours ⚬ Ideal slow-cooker size: 5- to 6-qt.

4 cups chicken broth

1 large boneless, skinless chicken breast

2 (15-oz.) cans black beans, rinsed and drained

16-oz. jar salsa

1 cup frozen corn

1 cup sliced fresh mushrooms

½ red onion, chopped

1 jalapeño pepper (whole)

1½ tsp. cumin

Salt and pepper to taste

Optional Toppings:

Shredded cheese

Sour cream

Cilantro

Avocado

1. Place all ingredients except the toppings in slow cooker. Stir.

2. Cover and cook on Low for 6–8 hours.

3. Remove the whole jalapeño.

4. Remove the chicken and shred between 2 forks. Replace back in the soup and stir.

5. Serve garnished with desired toppings.

Variation:

You may chop up the jalapeño for extra heat. Leaving it whole provides the flavor without the heat.

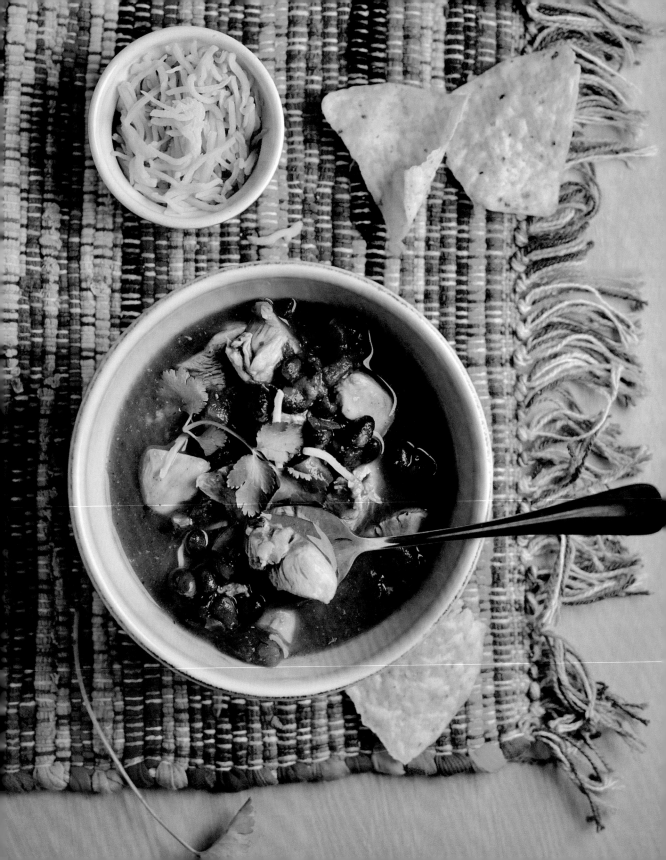

Easy Chicken Tortilla Soup

Becky Harder, Monument, CO

Makes 6–8 servings

Prep. Time: 5–10 minutes ⚭ *Cooking Time: 8 hours* ⚭ *Ideal slow-cooker size: 4- to 5-qt.*

4 chicken breast halves

2 (15-oz.) cans black beans, undrained

2 (15-oz.) cans Mexican stewed tomatoes, or Ro*Tel Diced Tomatoes and Green Chilies

1 cup salsa (mild, medium, or hot, whichever you prefer)

4-oz. can chopped green chiles

14½-oz. can tomato sauce

Tortilla chips

Shredded cheese

1. Combine all ingredients in large slow cooker.

2. Cover. Cook on Low for 8 hours.

3. Just before serving, remove chicken breasts and slice into bite-sized pieces. Stir into soup.

4. Put a handful of tortilla chips in each individual soup bowl. Ladle soup over chips. Top with shredded cheese.

SLOW COOKER

White Chicken Chili

Lucille Hollinger, Richland, PA

Makes 8 servings

Prep. Time: 10 minutes ⚬ *Cooking Time: 5–6 hours* ⚬ *Ideal slow-cooker size: 3-qt.*

4 cups cubed, cooked chicken

2 cups chicken broth

2 (14½-oz.) cans cannellini beans

14½-oz. can garbanzo beans

1 cup shredded white cheddar cheese

¼ cup chopped onion

¼ cup chopped bell pepper

2 tsp. ground cumin

½ tsp. dried oregano

¼ tsp. cayenne pepper

¼ tsp. salt

1. Combine all ingredients in slow cooker.

2. Cover and cook on Low for 5–6 hours.

Tip:

Serve with sour cream, shredded cheese, and tortilla chips.

Variation:

Omit garbanzo beans. Shred chicken instead of cubing it. Add 1 tsp. Italian herb seasoning.

—Beverly Hummel

Serving suggestion:

This chili is delicious with cornbread and salad.

Pork

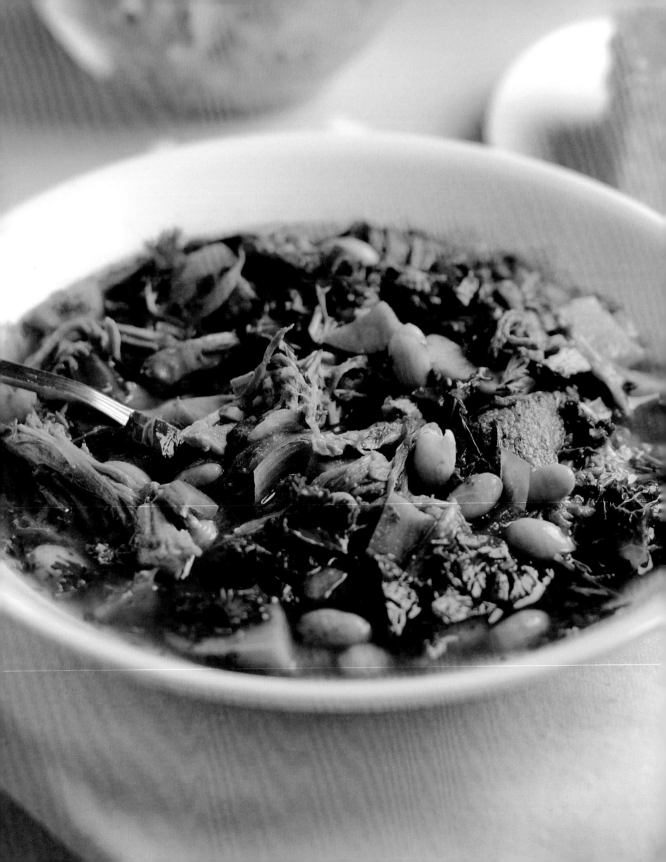

Italian Shredded Pork Stew

Emily Fox, Bernville, PA

Makes: 6–8 servings

Prep. Time: 20 minutes ⚘ *Cooking Time: 8–10 hours* ⚘ *Ideal slow-cooker size: 5-qt.*

2 medium sweet potatoes, peeled and cubed

2 cups chopped fresh kale

1 large onion, chopped

3 cloves garlic, minced

2½–3½ lb. boneless pork shoulder butt roast

14-oz. can white kidney or cannellini beans, drained

1½ tsp. Italian seasoning

½ tsp. salt

½ tsp. pepper

3 (14½-oz.) cans chicken broth

Sour cream, *optional*

1. Place sweet potatoes, kale, onion, and garlic in slow cooker.

2. Place roast on vegetables.

3. Add beans and seasonings.

4. Pour the broth over the other ingredients.

5. Cover and cook on Low for 8–10 hours or until meat is tender.

6. Remove meat. Skim fat from cooking juices if desired. Shred pork with 2 forks and return to cooker. Heat through.

7. Garnish with sour cream if desired.

DUTCH
OVEN

Italian Sausage Soup

Esther Porter, Minneapolis, MN

Makes 6–8 servings

Prep. Time: 15–25 minutes 🍃 Cooking Time: 65–70 minutes

1 lb. Italian sausage, casings removed

1 cup chopped onions

2 large cloves garlic, sliced

5 cups beef stock, or 3 (14½-oz.) cans beef broth

2 cups chopped or canned tomatoes

8-oz. can tomato sauce

1½ cups sliced zucchini

1 carrot, thinly sliced

1 medium-sized green bell pepper, diced

1 cup green beans, frozen or fresh

2 Tbsp. dried basil

2 Tbsp. dried oregano

8–10-oz. pkg. cheese tortellini

Salt and pepper to taste

Freshly grated Parmesan cheese for topping

1. Sauté sausage in heavy Dutch oven over medium heat until cooked through, about 10 minutes, breaking it up with a wooden spoon as it browns.

2. Using a slotted spoon, transfer sausage to a large bowl. Pour off all but 1 Tbsp. drippings from Dutch oven. Add onions and garlic to the 1 Tbsp. drippings and sauté until clear, about 5 minutes.

3. Return sausage to pan. Add beef stock, tomatoes, tomato sauce, zucchini, carrot, pepper, green beans, basil, and oregano. Simmer 30–40 minutes, or until vegetables are tender.

4. Add tortellini and cook 8–10 minutes. Season to taste with salt and pepper.

5. Ladle hot soup into bowls and sprinkle with Parmesan cheese.

Variations:

- You can use a large stockpot instead of a Dutch oven for this recipe.

- Use leftover meat and vegetables from your refrigerator, instead of the sausage and the vegetables listed above.

- Substitute V8 juice for half of the beef stock or tomatoes.

- When you're in a hurry, use Italian-style frozen vegetables instead of fresh beans, carrot, and zucchini.

Broccoli Rabe and Sausage Soup

Carlene Horne, Bedford, NH

Makes 4 servings

Prep. Time: 15 minutes ⚬ *Cooking Time: 15 minutes*

2 Tbsp. olive oil

1 onion, chopped

1 lb. sweet or spicy sausage, casing removed, sliced

1 bunch broccoli rabe, approximately 5 cups chopped

32 oz. chicken broth

1 cup water

8 oz. frozen tortellini

1. In a stockpot, heat the olive oil.

2. Add the onion and sausage and sauté until tender.

3. Add the broccoli rabe and sauté for a few more minutes.

4. Pour the broth and water into the stockpot pan; bring to a simmer.

5. Add the tortellini and cook a few minutes until tender.

Tip:

Substitute any green, such as Swiss chard, kale, or spinach, for the broccoli rabe.

Serving suggestion:

Serve with grated cheese and crusty bread.

Hearty Lentil and Sausage Stew

Cindy Krestynick, Glen Lyon, PA

Makes 6 servings

Prep. Time: 5–10 minutes ♣ *Cooking Time: 4–6 hours* ♣ *Ideal slow-cooker size: 6-qt.*

2 cups dried lentils, picked over and rinsed

14½-oz. can diced tomatoes

8 cups canned chicken broth, or water

1 Tbsp. salt

½–1 lb. pork or beef sausage, cut into 2-inch pieces

1. In a slow cooker, stir the lentils, tomatoes, chicken broth, and salt to combine. Place the sausage pieces on top.

2. Cover and cook on Low for 4–6 hours, or until the lentils are tender but not dry or mushy.

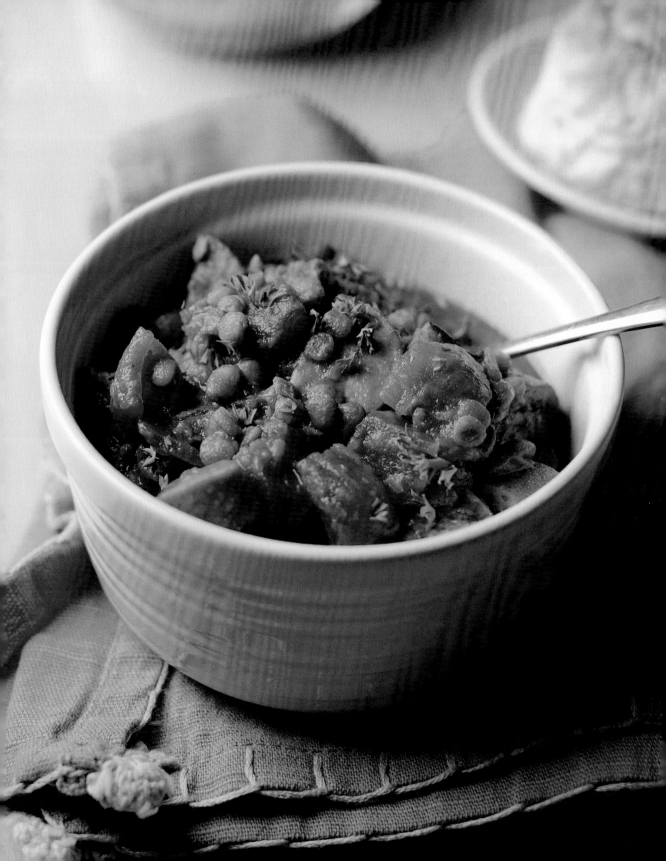

Kale Chowder

Colleen Heatwole, Burton, MI

Makes 8 servings

Prep. Time: 30 minutes ⚜ *Cooking Time: 6 hours* ⚜ *Ideal slow-cooker size: 6-qt.*

8 cups chicken broth

1 bunch of kale, cleaned, stems removed, chopped

2 lb. potatoes, peeled and diced

4 cloves garlic, minced

1 medium onion, diced

1 lb. cooked ham

½ tsp. pepper, or to taste

1. Combine all ingredients in slow cooker.

2. Cover and cook on Low for 6 hours or until vegetables are tender.

Tip:

If you have "new" potatoes, peeling is optional.

Split Pea Soup

SLOW COOKER

Kelly Amos, Pittsboro, NC

Makes 8 servings

Prep. Time: 10 minutes ⚓ *Cooking Time: 8–9 hours* ⚓ *Ideal slow-cooker size: 4½-qt.*

2 cups dried split peas

8 cups water

2 onions, chopped

2 carrots, peeled and sliced

4 slices Canadian bacon, chopped

2 Tbsp. chicken bouillon granules,
or 2 chicken bouillon cubes

1 tsp. salt

¼–½ tsp. pepper

1. Combine all ingredients in slow cooker.

2. Cover. Cook on Low for 8–9 hours.

Variation:

For a creamier soup, remove half of the soup when done and puree. Stir back into rest of soup.

Beef

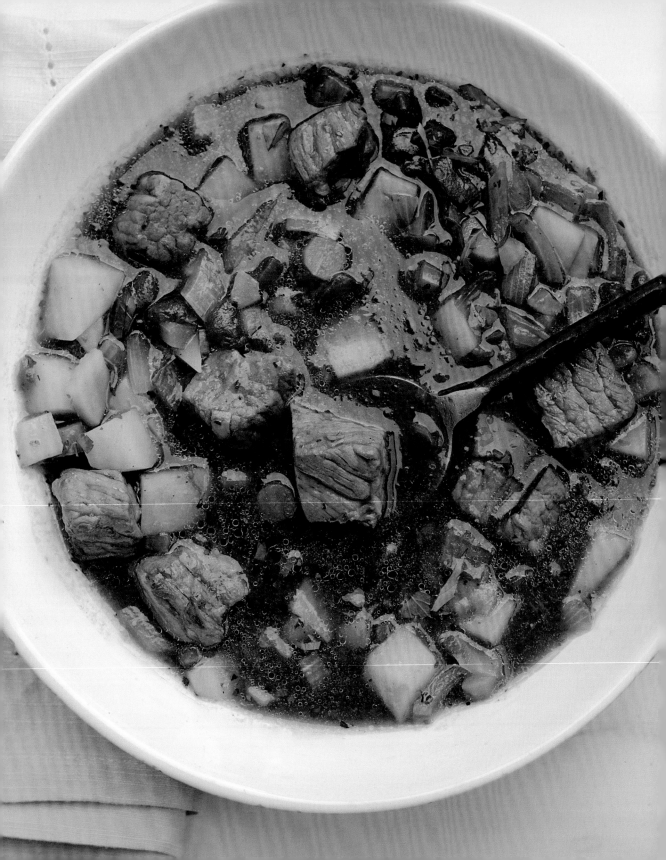

Beef Vegetable Soup

Margaret Moffitt, Bartlett, TN

Makes 12 servings

Prep. Time: 15 minutes ❧ *Cooking Time: 6–8 hours* ❧ *Ideal slow-cooker size: 4-qt.*

1 lb. stewing beef chunks

28-oz. can stewed tomatoes, undrained

28-oz. water (use empty tomato can)

16-oz. pkg. your favorite frozen vegetable

5 ounces frozen chopped onions

1½ tsp. salt

¼–½ tsp. pepper

2 Tbsp. chopped fresh parsley, *optional*

1. In a slow cooker, combine all the ingredients.

2. Cover and cook on High for 6–8 hours.

SLOW COOKER

Minestrone Soup

Dorothy Shank, Sterling, IL

Makes 8 servings

Prep. Time: 10 minutes   ⚬   Cooking Time: 4–12 hours   ⚬   Ideal slow-cooker size: 4- to 5-qt.

3 cups beef stock

1½ lb. stewing meat, cut into bite-sized pieces

1 medium onion, diced

4 carrots, diced

14½-oz. can diced tomatoes

1 tsp. salt

10-oz. pkg. frozen mixed vegetables, or your choice of frozen vegetables

1 Tbsp. dried basil

½ cup dry elbow noodles, vermicelli, or other pasta

1 tsp. dried oregano

1. Combine all ingredients in slow cooker. Stir well.

2. Cover. Cook on Low for 10–12 hours, or on High for 4–5 hours.

Serving suggestion:
Top individual servings with grated Parmesan cheese.

Italian Pasta Soup

Sharon Timpe, Jackson, WI

Makes 6 servings

Prep. Time: 10–15 minutes ⚭ *Cooking Time: 30 minutes*

2 (14½-oz.) cans chicken broth

1 cup water

1 cup uncooked elbow macaroni

18 frozen Italian-style or regular meatballs

2 cups fresh spinach leaves, finely shredded

8-oz. can pizza sauce

1. In a large stockpot, bring the broth and the water to a boil.

2. Add the pasta and meatballs and return to a boil. Lower the heat and continue cooking for 8–10 minutes, or until the pasta is done and the meatballs are hot. Stir occasionally. Do not drain.

3. Add the spinach and pizza sauce. Simmer for 2 minutes, or until heated thoroughly.

STOVETOP

Pasta Fagioli

Stacie Skelly, Millersville, PA

Makes 8–10 servings

Prep. Time: 20 minutes ⚘ *Cooking Time: 1½ hours*

1 lb. ground beef
1 cup diced onions
1 cup julienned carrots
1 cup chopped celery
2 cloves garlic, minced
2 (14½-oz.) cans diced
  tomatoes, undrained
15-oz. can red kidney beans, undrained
15-oz. can great northern
  beans, undrained
15-oz. can tomato sauce
12-oz. can V8 juice
1 Tbsp. vinegar
1½ tsp. salt
1 tsp. dried oregano
1 tsp. dried basil
½ tsp. pepper
½ tsp. dried thyme
½ lb. ditali pasta

1. Brown ground beef in a large stockpot. Drain off drippings.

2. To browned beef, add onions, carrots, celery, and garlic. Sauté for 10 minutes.

3. Add remaining ingredients, except pasta, and stir well. Simmer, covered, for 1 hour.

4. About 50 minutes into cooking time, cook pasta in a separate saucepan, according to the directions on the package.

5. Add drained pasta to the large pot of soup. Simmer for 5–10 minutes and serve.

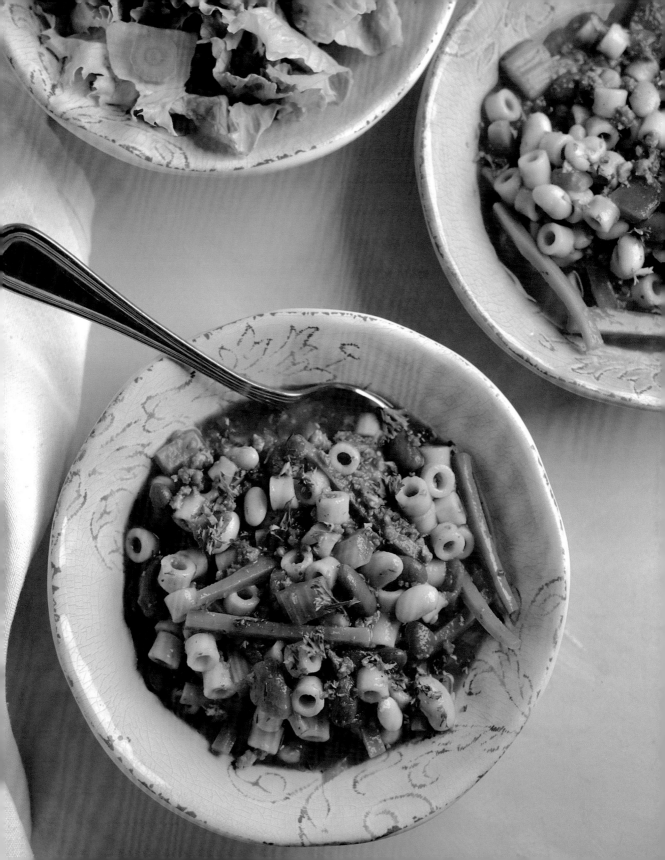

Hearty Beef Barley Soup

Karen Gingrich, New Holland, PA

Makes 4–5 servings

Prep. Time: 5–10 minutes & Cooking Time: 35 minutes

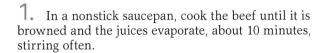

1 lb. beef tips
2 cups sliced fresh mushrooms
¼ tsp. garlic powder
32-oz. can (3½ cups) beef broth
2 medium carrots, sliced
¼ tsp. dried thyme
Dash pepper
½ cup quick-cooking barley

1. In a nonstick saucepan, cook the beef until it is browned and the juices evaporate, about 10 minutes, stirring often.

2. Add the mushrooms and garlic powder and cook until the mushrooms begin to wilt, about 5 minutes.

3. Add the broth, carrots, thyme, and pepper.

4. Heat to a boil. Stir in the barley. Cover and cook over low heat for 20 minutes, or until the barley is tender.

Instantly Good Beef Stew

Hope Comerford, Clinton Township, MI

Makes 6 servings

Prep. Time: 20 minutes   ☆   Cooking Time: 35 minutes

3 Tbsp. olive oil

2 lb. stewing beef, cubed

2 cloves garlic, minced

1 large onion, chopped

3 celery stalks, sliced

3 large potatoes, cubed

2–3 carrots, sliced

8 oz. no-salt-added tomato sauce

10 oz. low-sodium beef broth

2 tsp. Worcestershire sauce

¼ tsp. pepper

1 bay leaf

1. Set the Instant Pot to the Sauté function, then add 1 Tbsp. of the oil. Add ⅓ of the beef cubes and brown and sear all sides. Repeat this process twice more with the remaining oil and beef cubes. Set the beef aside.

2. Place the garlic, onion, and celery into the pot and sauté for a few minutes. Press Cancel.

3. Add the beef back in as well as all the remaining ingredients.

4. Secure the lid and make sure the vent is set to sealing. Choose Manual for 35 minutes.

5. When cook time is up, let the pressure release naturally for 15 minutes, then release any remaining pressure manually.

6. Remove the lid, remove the bay leaf, then serve.

Note:

If you want your stew to be a bit thicker, remove some of the potatoes, mash, then stir them back through the stew.

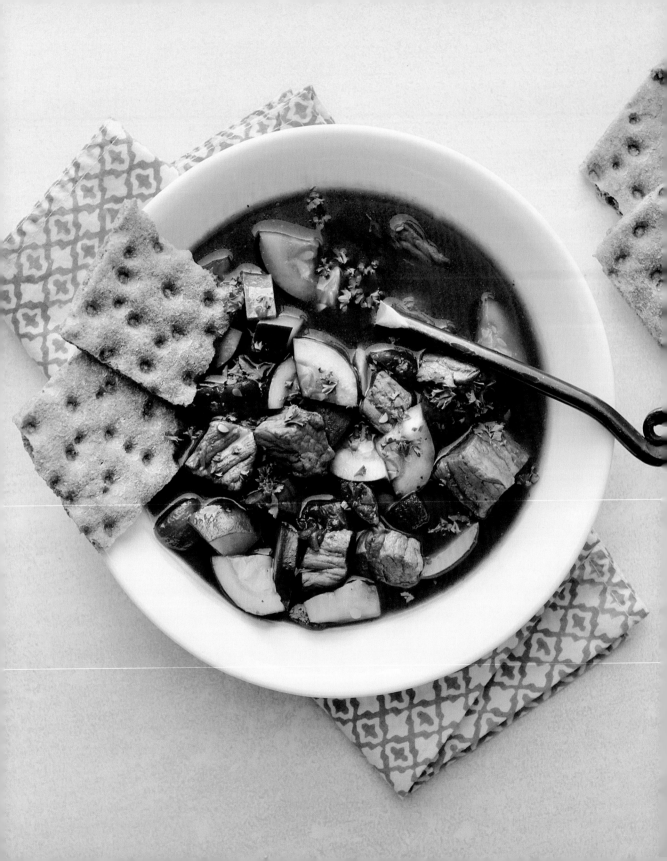

Mediterranean Beef Stew

SLOW COOKER

Sandy Osborn, Iowa City, IA

Makes 4 servings

Prep. Time: 5–10 minutes ⚬ *Cooking Time: 3–8 hours* ⚬ *Ideal slow-cooker size: 3½-qt.*

2 medium zucchini, cut into bite-sized pieces

¾ lb. beef stew meat, cut into ½-inch pieces

2 (14½-oz.) cans Italian-style diced tomatoes, undrained

½ tsp. pepper, *optional*

2-inch stick cinnamon, or ¼ tsp. ground cinnamon

1. Place the zucchini in the bottom of a slow cooker.

2. Add the beef and remaining ingredients in the order they are listed.

3. Cover and cook on High for 3–5 hours, or until the meat is tender but not overcooked. You can also cook the stew on High for 1 hour, then on Low for 7 hours, or until the meat is tender but not overdone. Remove the cinnamon stick before serving.

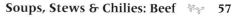

Tuscan Beef Stew

Orpha Herr, Andover, NY

Makes 12 servings

Prep. Time: 20 minutes ❧ Cooking Time: 8½–9½ hours ❧ Ideal slow-cooker size: 6-qt.

10¾-oz. can tomato soup

1½ cups beef broth

½ cup burgundy wine or
other red wine

1 tsp. Italian herb seasoning

½ tsp. garlic powder

14½-oz. can diced Italian-style
tomatoes, undrained

½ cup diced onion

3 large carrots, cut in 1-inch pieces

2 lb. stew beef, cut into 1-inch pieces

2 (16-oz.) cans cannellini beans,
rinsed and drained

1. Stir soup, broth, wine, Italian seasoning, garlic powder, tomatoes, onion, carrots, and beef into slow cooker.

2. Cover and cook on Low for 8–9 hours or until vegetables are tender-crisp.

3. Stir in beans. Turn to High until heated through, 10–20 minutes more.

Chunky Beef Chili

Ruth C. Hancock, Earlsboro, OK

Makes 4 servings

Prep. Time: 30 minutes   *Cooking Time: 1¾–2¼ hours*

2 Tbsp. vegetable oil, *divided*

1 lb. beef stew, cut into 1½-inch thick pieces

1 medium onion, chopped

1 medium jalapeño pepper with seeds, minced, *optional*

½ tsp. salt

2 (14½-oz.) cans chili-seasoned diced tomatoes

1. Heat 1 Tbsp. oil in stockpot over medium heat until hot.

2. Brown half of beef in oil. Remove meat from pot and keep warm.

3. Repeat with remaining beef. Remove meat from pot and keep warm.

4. Add remaining 1 Tbsp. oil to stockpot, along with the onion, and the pepper if you wish.

5. Cook 5–8 minutes, or until vegetables are tender. Stir occasionally.

6. Return meat and juices to stockpot. Add salt and tomatoes.

7. Bring to a boil. Reduce heat. Cover tightly and simmer 1¾–2¼ hours, or until meat is tender but not dried out.

INSTANT POT

Chili Comerford Style

Hope Comerford, Clinton Township, MI

Makes 4–6 servings

Prep. Time: 10 minutes   Cooking Time: 15 minutes

1 tsp. olive oil

1 lb. ground round

1 medium onion, chopped

15½-oz. can kidney beans, rinsed and drained

2 (14½-oz.) cans diced tomatoes

10-oz. can cream of tomato soup (I use Pacific Foods Creamy Tomato)

3 cloves garlic, minced

2 tsp. tarragon

1 tsp. salt

1 tsp. pepper

2 tsp. chili powder

1 cup beef stock

3–6 cups water, depending on how thick or thin you like your chili

1. Set the Instant Pot to the Sauté function and let it get hot. Pour in the olive oil and coat the bottom of the pot.

2. Brown the ground round with the onion. This will take about 5–7 minutes.

3. Press Cancel. Carefully drain the grease.

4. Place the remaining ingredients into the inner pot with the beef and onion.

5. Secure the lid and set the vent to sealing. Manually set the cook time for 15 minutes on high pressure.

6. When cook time is up, manually release the pressure. When the pin drops, remove the lid and serve.

Serving suggestion:

We love to add a dollop of sour cream and a bit of shredded sharp cheddar to our chili.

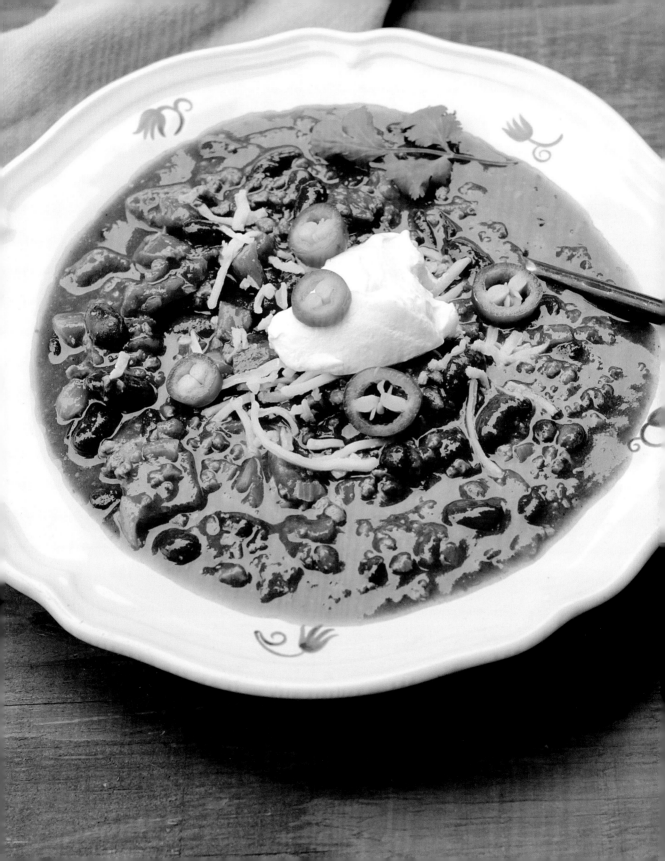

Meatless

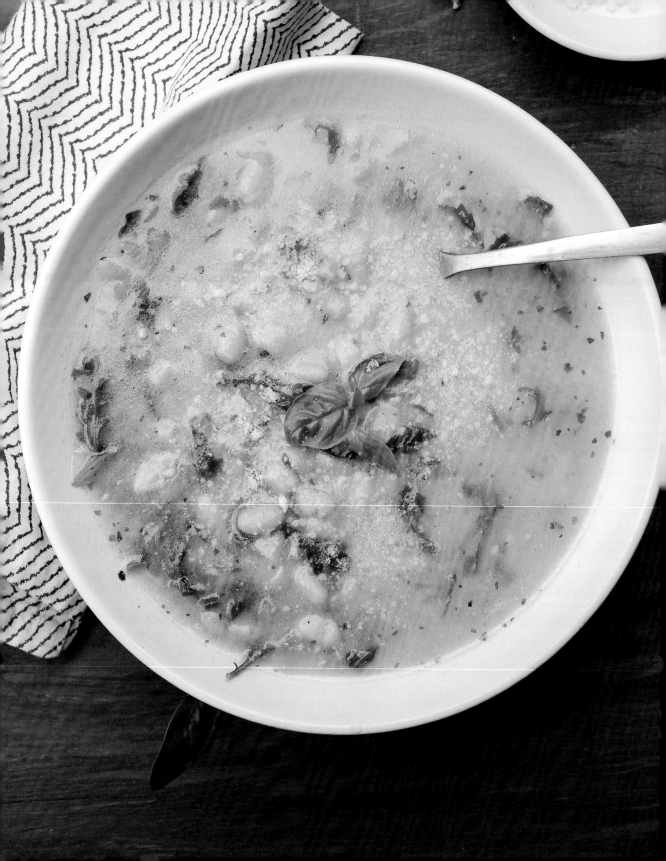

Cannellini Bean Soup

Hope Comerford, Clinton Township, MI

Makes 6–8 servings

Prep. Time: 10 minutes & Soaking Time: overnight & Cooking Time: 30 minutes

2 Tbsp. extra-virgin olive oil

4 cloves garlic, sliced very thin

1 small onion, chopped

2 heads escarole, well washed and cut medium-fine (about 8 cups)

8-oz. bag dried cannellini beans, soaked overnight

8 cups low-sodium vegetable stock

3 basil leaves, chopped fine

Parmesan cheese shavings, *optional*

Tip:

If you do not remember to soak the beans overnight, or if you don't have time to soak them, simply cook the soup on high pressure for 51 minutes instead.

1. Set the Instant Pot to Sauté and heat the olive oil.

2. Sauté the garlic, onion, and escarole until the onion is translucent.

3. Hit the Cancel button on your Instant Pot and add the beans and stock.

4. Secure the lid and set the vent to sealing.

5. Manually set the time for 25 minutes on high pressure.

6. When the cooking time is over, let the pressure release naturally. Remove the lid when the pin drops and spoon into serving bowls.

7. Top each bowl with a sprinkle of the chopped basil leaves and a few Parmesan shavings (if using).

Chipotle Navy Bean Soup

Rebecca Weybright, Manheim, PA

Makes 6 servings

Prep. Time: 10 minutes ⚘ *Cooking Time: 8 hours*
Soaking Time: 8–12 hours ⚘ *Ideal slow-cooker size: 5-qt.*

1½ cups dried navy beans

1 onion, chopped

1 dried chipotle chili, soaked 10–15 minutes in cold water

4 cups water

1–2 tsp. salt

2 cups canned tomatoes with juice

1. Soak the beans overnight (8–12 hours). Drain and rinse the soaked beans.

2. Add to slow cooker with onion, chili, and water.

3. Cover and cook on Low for 8 hours until beans are creamy.

4. Add salt and tomatoes.

5. If desired, use an immersion blender to puree soup.

Black Bean Chili

SLOW COOKER

Joyce Cox, Port Angeles, WA

Makes 8 servings

Prep. Time: 20 minutes ❧ *Cooking Time: 6–8 hours* ❧ *Ideal slow-cooker size: 6-qt.*

1½ cups fresh-brewed coffee

1½ cups vegetable broth

2 (15-oz.) cans diced tomatoes with juice

15-oz. can tomato sauce

8 cups cooked black beans, drained

1 medium yellow onion, diced

4 cloves garlic, minced

2 Tbsp. brown sugar, packed

2 Tbsp. chili powder

1 Tbsp. ground cumin

Salt to taste

1. Combine all ingredients except salt in slow cooker.

2. Cover and cook on Low for 6–8 hours. Add salt near end of cooking.

Tip:

Great served in bowls with cilantro, cubed avocados, Greek yogurt or sour cream, and grated cheese on top.

Variation:

Use 4 (15-oz.) cans of black beans, rinsed and drained, instead of the 8 cups cooked black beans. Mash some of the beans with a potato masher before adding to cooker. The chili will be thicker.

Summer Chili

Hope Comerford, Clinton Township, MI

Makes 6 servings

Prep. Time: 15 minutes ⚮ *Cooking Time: 3½–4 hours* ⚮ *Ideal slow-cooker size: 3-qt.*

28-oz. can Red Gold sliced tomatoes and zucchini

15-oz. can tomato sauce

14-oz. can petite diced tomatoes with green chiles

15½-oz. can chili beans

15¼-oz. can black beans, rinsed and drained

1 medium onion, roughly chopped

3 small yellow squash, halved, quartered, and chopped

3 Tbsp. garlic powder

2 Tbsp. onion powder

1 tsp. salt

⅛ tsp. pepper

2 cups water

1. Place all ingredients into the crock and stir.

2. Cover and cook on Low for 3½–4 hours.

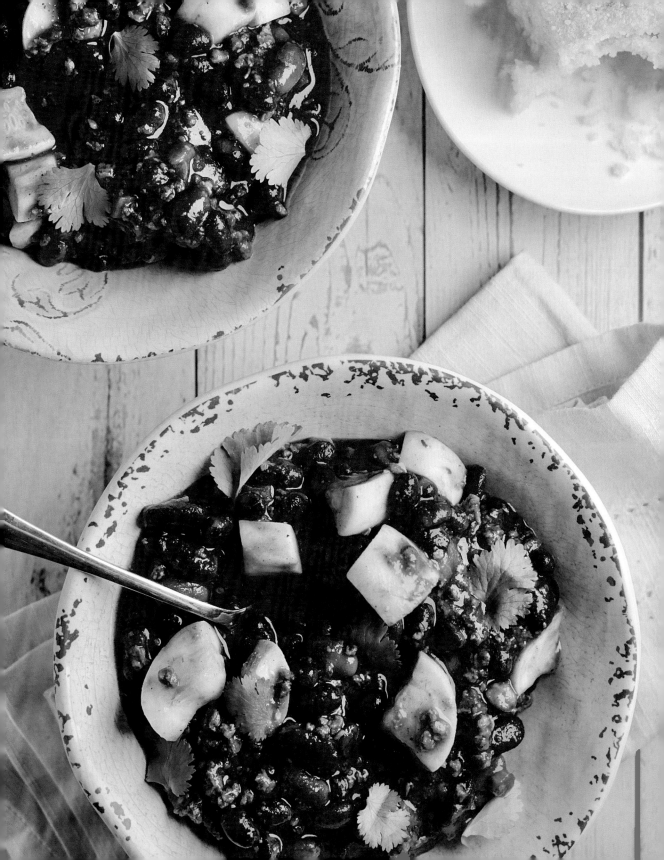

Red Lentil Soup

Carolyn Spohn, Shawnee, KS

Makes 4–6 servings

Prep. Time: 20 minutes ❧ *Cooking Time: 3–4 hours* ❧ *Ideal slow-cooker size: 5-qt.*

¾ cup dried red lentils

½ cup brown rice, uncooked

4 cups vegetable broth

1 small potato, diced

2 medium carrots, chopped

1 small onion, chopped

2 cloves garlic, chopped

½ tsp. turmeric

¼ tsp. ground cumin

¼ tsp. ground coriander

Salt and pepper to taste

Plain yogurt, for serving

1. Combine all ingredients except plain yogurt in slow cooker.

2. Cover and cook on High for 3–4 hours, until vegetables are soft.

3. Puree with immersion blender until smooth.

4. Serve in bowls with a little plain yogurt dolloped on top.

Tip:

Other orange-colored vegetables can be used with or instead of carrots. Red or orange sweet peppers and/or butternut squash are good. This is a very flexible soup, as you can vary the vegetables according to what you have on hand.

Serving suggestion:

Sprinkle with chopped cilantro.

Sweet Potato Lentil Soup

Joleen Albrecht, Gladstone, MI

Makes 6 servings

Prep. Time: 10–15 minutes   *Cooking Time: 6 hours*   *Ideal slow-cooker size: 4-qt.*

4 cups vegetable broth

3 cups (about 1 ¼ lb.) peeled and cubed sweet potatoes

3 medium carrots, chopped

1 medium onion, chopped

4 cloves garlic, minced

1 cup dried lentils, rinsed

½ tsp. ground cumin

¼ tsp. salt

¼ tsp. cayenne pepper

¼ tsp. ground ginger

¼ cup minced fresh cilantro or 1–2 Tbsp. dried cilantro

1. Combine all ingredients in slow cooker.

2. Cover. Cook on Low for 6 hours, or until vegetables are done to your liking.

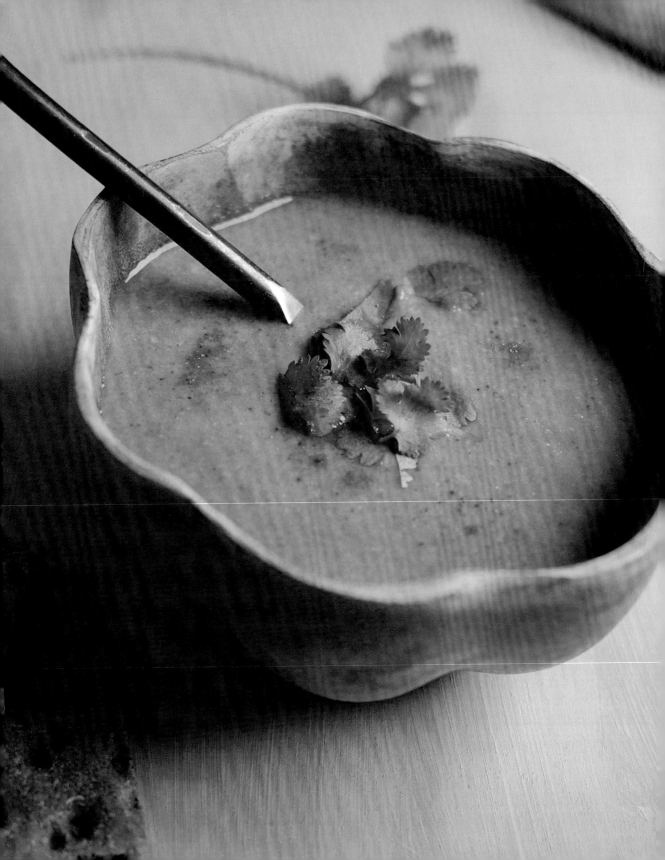

Coconut-Curried Spinach Pea Soup

Allison Martin, Royal Oak, MI

Makes 12 servings

Prep. Time: 45 minutes ⚶ *Cooking Time: 7–8 hours* ⚶ *Ideal slow-cooker size: 5-qt.*

5 cups water

2 tsp. salt

8 cloves garlic, peeled

4 cups diced sweet potatoes, peeled or unpeeled

1 Tbsp. coconut oil

4 cups chopped onions

1½ tsp. ginger

1½ tsp. turmeric

1½ tsp. cumin

1½ tsp. coriander

½ tsp. cinnamon

½ tsp. cardamom

¼–½ tsp. cayenne, according to your taste preference

Black pepper to taste

1½ Tbsp. lemon juice

3 cups frozen peas

4 cups torn fresh spinach

14-oz. can low-fat coconut milk

1. Combine all ingredients in your crock and mix well.

2. Cover and cook on Low for 7–8 hours, or until the potatoes are tender when poked with a fork.

3. Puree soup with an immersion blender or a potato masher until as smooth as you like.

Serving suggestion:

Serve with an optional garnish of fresh cilantro and/or a dollop of nonfat plain Greek yogurt on top.

Wild Rice Mushroom Soup

Kelly Amos, Pittsboro, NC

Makes 4 servings

Prep. Time: 15–20 minutes ❧ *Cooking Time: 35 minutes*

1 Tbsp. olive oil

½ white onion, chopped

¼ cup chopped celery

¼ cup chopped carrots

1½ cups sliced fresh white mushrooms

½ cup white wine, or ½ cup low-sodium, fat-free chicken broth

2½ cups low-sodium, fat-free chicken broth

1 cup fat-free half-and-half

2 Tbsp. flour

¼ tsp. dried thyme

Black pepper to taste

1 cup cooked wild rice

1. Put olive oil in stockpot and heat. Carefully add chopped onion, celery, and carrots. Cook until tender.

2. Add mushrooms, white wine, and chicken broth.

3. Cover and heat through.

4. In a bowl, blend half-and-half, flour, thyme, and pepper. Then stir in cooked wild rice.

5. Pour rice mixture into hot stockpot with vegetables.

6. Cook over medium heat. Stir continually until thickened and bubbly.

Main Dishes

Chicken & Turkey

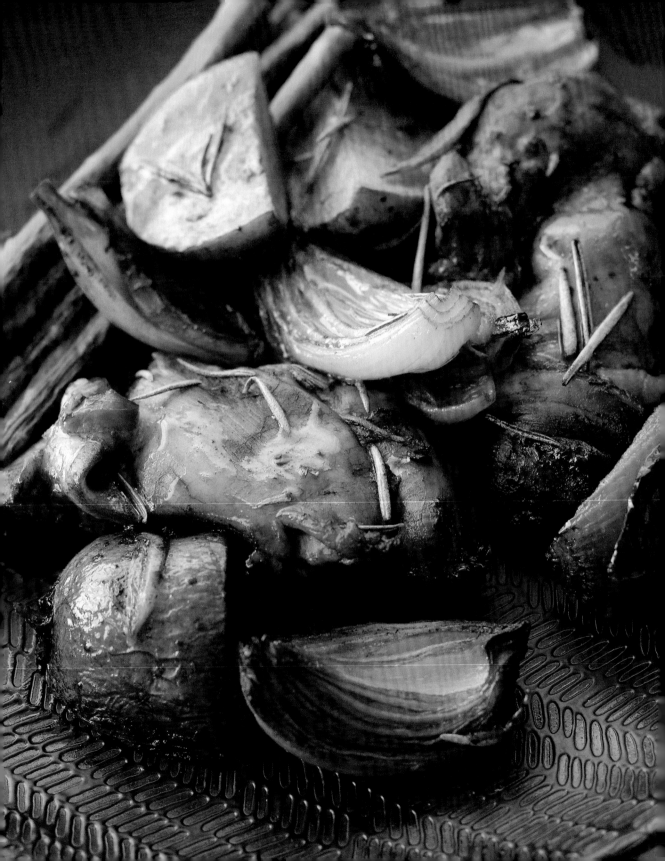

Chicken Baked with Red Onions, Potatoes, and Parsley

OVEN

Kristine Stalter, Iowa City, IA

Makes 8 servings

Prep. Time: 10–15 minutes ⚬ Baking Time: 45–60 minutes

2 red onions, each cut into 10 wedges

1¼ lb. new potatoes, unpeeled and cut into chunks

2 garlic bulbs, separated into cloves, unpeeled

Salt and pepper to taste

3 tsp. extra-virgin olive oil

2 Tbsp. balsamic vinegar

5 sprigs rosemary

8 chicken thighs, skin removed

1. Spread the onions, potatoes, and garlic in single layer over the bottom of a large roasting pan so that they will crisp and brown.

2. Season with salt and pepper.

3. Pour over the oil and balsamic vinegar and add rosemary, leaving some sprigs whole and stripping the leaves off the rest.

4. Toss the vegetables and seasonings together.

5. Tuck the chicken pieces among the vegetables.

6. Bake at 400°F for 45–60 minutes, or until the chicken and vegetables are cooked through.

7. Transfer to a big platter or take to the table in the roasting pan.

GRILL

Sizzlin' Chicken Skewers

Cheryl A. Lapp, Parkesburg, PA

Makes 6 servings

Prep. Time: 30 minutes ❧ *Marinating Time: 1½ hours* ❧ *Grilling or Broiling Time: 12 minutes*

⅓ cup hot water

¼ cup barbecue sauce

¼ cup creamy peanut butter

¼ cup soy sauce

2 Tbsp. honey Dijon mustard

1 lb. boneless, skinless chicken breasts, cut into small pieces

1 red pepper, cut into chunks

1 yellow pepper, cut into chunks

2 (15-oz.) cans whole potatoes

20-oz. can pineapple chunks

1 small zucchini, cut into chunks

1. In a small mixing bowl, combine first five ingredients. Brush small amount onto chicken pieces, enough to cover. Let stand for 1½ hours.

2. Alternate chicken and vegetables and pineapple chunks on skewers and brush with remaining sauce.

3. Place skewers on the grill for approximately 6 minutes. Turn and grill another 6 minutes.

Variation:

You can cook these under the broiler instead. Place them under the broiler for 6 minutes, then turn and broil for another 6 minutes.

Lemon-Chicken Oven Bake

Judi Manos, West Islip, NY

Makes 4 servings

Prep. Time: 10–15 minutes ⚘ *Baking Time: 45–50 minutes*

¼ cup zesty Italian dressing

½ cup chicken broth

1 Tbsp. honey

1½ lb. bone-in chicken legs and thighs

1 lb. new potatoes, quartered

5 cloves garlic, peeled

1 lemon, cut in 8 wedges

1 tsp. dried rosemary, *optional*

1. In a mixing bowl, blend together Italian dressing, broth, and honey.

2. Arrange chicken, potatoes, and garlic in well-greased 9 × 13-inch baking dish.

3. Drizzle with dressing mixture.

4. Situate lemons and rosemary, if using, among the chicken and potatoes.

5. Bake at 400°F for 45–50 minutes, or until chicken is done and potatoes are tender. (Temperature probe inserted into center of chicken should register 165°F.)

Chicken Dinner in a Packet

Bonnie Whaling, Clearfield, PA

Makes 4 servings

Prep. Time: 25 minutes   Baking Time: 30–35 minutes

4 (5-oz.) boneless skinless chicken breast halves

2 cups sliced fresh mushrooms

2 medium carrots, cut in thin strips, about 1 cup

1 medium zucchini, unpeeled and sliced, about 1½ cups

2 Tbsp. olive, or canola, oil

2 Tbsp. lemon juice

4 tsp. fresh basil, or 1 tsp. dried basil

¼ tsp. salt

¼ tsp. black pepper

1. Preheat oven to 375°F.

2. Fold four 12 × 28-inch pieces of foil in half to make four 12 × 14-inch rectangles. Place one chicken breast half on each piece of foil.

3. Top with mushrooms, carrots, and zucchini, dividing vegetables equally among chicken bundles.

4. In a small bowl, stir together oil, lemon juice, basil, salt, and pepper.

5. Drizzle oil mixture over vegetables and chicken.

6. Pull up two opposite edges of foil. Seal with a double fold. Then fold in remaining edges, leaving enough space for steam to build.

7. Place bundles side-by-side in a shallow baking pan.

8. Bake 30–35 minutes, or until chicken reaches 170°F on an instant-read thermometer.

9. Serve dinners in foil packets, or transfer to serving plate.

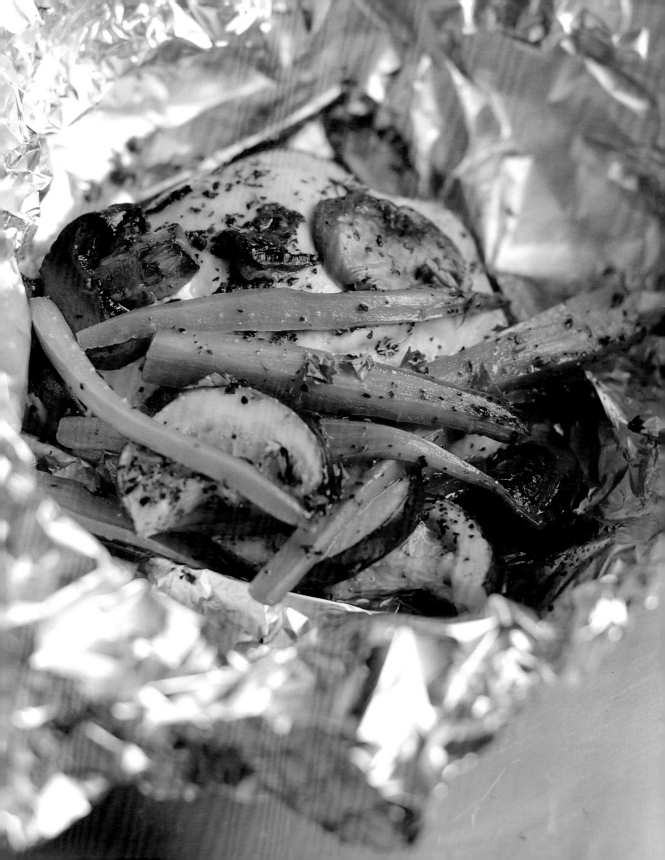

Lemon Pepper Chicken with Veggies

Nadine Martinitz, Salina, KS

Makes 4 servings

Prep. Time: 20 minutes ❧ *Cooking Time: 4–10 hours* ❧ *Ideal slow-cooker size: 4-qt.*

4 carrots, sliced ½-inch thick

4 potatoes, cut in 1-inch chunks

2 cloves garlic, peeled and minced, *optional*

4 whole chicken legs and thighs, skin removed

2 tsp. lemon pepper seasoning

Poultry seasoning, *optional*

1¾ cup low-sodium, gluten-free chicken broth

1. Layer vegetables and chicken in slow cooker.

2. Sprinkle with lemon pepper seasoning and poultry seasoning if you wish. Pour broth over all.

3. Cover and cook on Low for 8–10 hours or on High for 4–5 hours.

Variation:

Add 2 cups frozen green beans to the bottom layer in the cooker.

—Earnest Zimmerman

Chicken Bruschetta Bake

OVEN

Krista Hershberger, Elverson, PA

Makes 6 servings

Prep. Time: 15 minutes   *Baking Time: 60 minutes*

1½ lb. boneless, skinless chicken breasts, cut into cubes

1 tsp. Italian seasoning

28-oz. can Italian-style stewed tomatoes, well drained

¾ cup shredded mozzarella cheese

6-oz. pkg. stuffing mix for chicken

1½ cups water

1. Place the chicken in a lightly greased 9 × 13-inch baking dish. Sprinkle with the Italian seasoning.

2. Spread the tomatoes over the top.

3. Sprinkle with the cheese.

4. In a mixing bowl, combine the stuffing mix with the water. Spoon over the ingredients in the baking dish.

5. Cover and bake for 30 minutes. Remove cover and bake for 30 more minutes

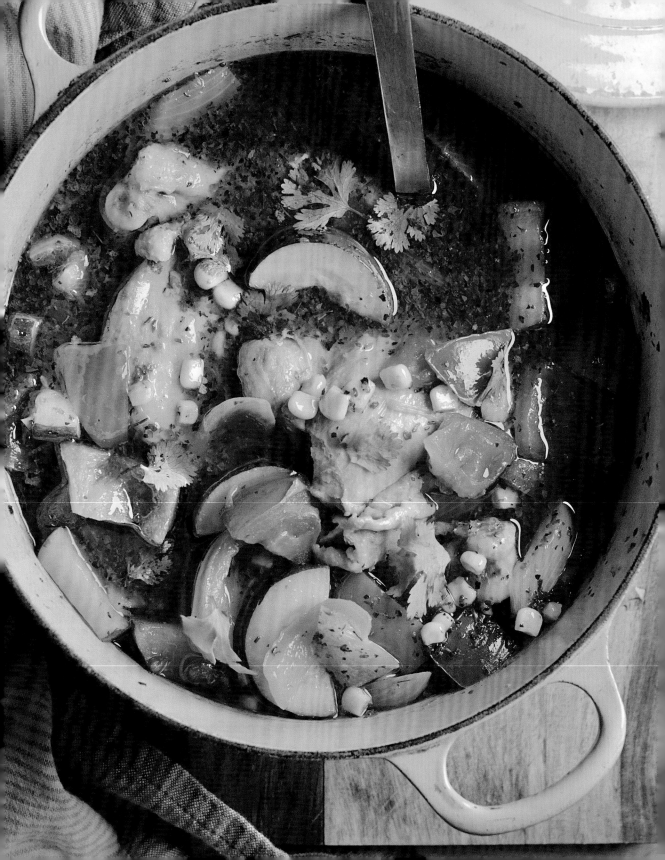

Chicken Recuerdos de Tucson

DUTCH OVEN

Joanna Harrison, Lafayette, CO

Makes 6 servings

Prep. Time: 15 minutes ⚬ Cooking Time: 30–40 minutes

I whole chicken, cut up, or 6 chicken legs and thighs

I Tbsp. olive oil

I medium onion, chopped coarsely

3 cloves garlic, minced

I tsp. ground cumin

2–3 green chiles, chopped, according to your taste preference

I green bell pepper, chopped

1–2 zucchini, sliced

I cup chopped tomatoes

2 cups corn

2 tsp. oregano

I tsp. basil

2 cups chicken broth

Cilantro for garnish

1. Brown chicken in olive oil in Dutch oven. Remove chicken to platter. Reserve pan drippings.

2. Gently sauté onion and garlic in drippings until wilted.

3. Stir in cumin, green chiles, green pepper, and zucchini. Sauté until peppers wilt.

4. Add tomatoes, corn, oregano, basil, and broth.

5. Return chicken to pot.

6. Cover. Simmer 30–40 minutes, or until chicken is tender to the bone.

7. Garnish with cilantro and serve.

Variation:

You can cook this in a large stockpot instead.

Easy Chicken Fajitas

Jessica Hontz, Coatesville, PA

Makes 4–6 servings

Prep. Time: 20 minutes   ❧   *Marinating Time: 4–8 hours, or overnight*   ❧   *Cooking Time: 10 minutes*

1 lb. boneless, skinless chicken breasts

0.7-oz. pkg. dry Italian salad dressing mix

8-oz. bottle Italian salad dressing

1 cup salsa

1 green pepper, sliced

½ medium-sized onion, sliced

10 (10-inch) flour tortillas

Optional Toppings:

Shredded Monterey Jack cheese

Shredded lettuce

Sour cream

Chopped tomatoes

Salsa

Hot pepper sauce

1. Cut chicken into thin strips. Place in large mixing bowl.

2. Add dry salad dressing mix and salad dressing. Mix well. Cover and marinade 4–8 hours in the fridge.

3. In a large skillet, combine drained chicken strips, salsa, and pepper and onion slices. Stir-fry until chicken is cooked and peppers and onions are soft.

4. Place chicken mix in tortillas with your choice of toppings.

Variation:

The cooked chicken can also be used on salads.

Chicken and Broccoli Bake

Jan Rankin, Millersville, PA

Makes 12–16 servings

Prep. Time: 15 minutes   *Baking Time: 30 minutes*

2 (10¾-oz.) cans cream of chicken soup

2½ cups milk, *divided*

16-oz. bag frozen chopped broccoli, thawed and drained

3 cups cooked, chopped chicken breast

2 cups buttermilk baking mix

1. In a large mixing bowl, mix the soup and 1 cup milk together until smooth.

2. Stir in the broccoli and chicken.

3. Pour into a well-greased 9 × 13-inch baking dish.

4. In a mixing bowl, combine 1½ cups milk and the baking mix.

5. Spoon the baking mixture evenly over the top of the chicken-broccoli mixture.

6. Bake at 450°F for 30 minutes.

Simmering Chicken Dinner

Trish Dick, Ladysmith, WI

Makes 4 servings

Prep. Time: 10 minutes  *Cooking Time: 40 minutes*

2½ cups chicken broth

½ cup apple juice

1 bay leaf

½ tsp. garlic powder

½ tsp. paprika

¼ tsp. salt

1½ lb. boneless, skinless chicken breasts, or thighs, cut into chunks

1 cup uncooked whole grain rice

3 cups fresh, or frozen, vegetables: your choice of one, or a mix

Additional ½ tsp. paprika, *optional*

Parsley as garnish, *optional*

1. Heat chicken broth, apple juice, bay leaf, garlic powder, paprika, and salt in large skillet until boiling, stirring occasionally.

2. Add chicken. Cover. Reduce heat and simmer 10 minutes on low.

3. Turn chicken.

4. Add 1 cup rice around chicken.

5. Top with the vegetables.

6. Cover. Simmer 25 minutes, or until rice is cooked, vegetables are as soft as you like, and chicken is done.

7. Remove bay leaf.

8. Sprinkle with paprika and parsley before serving if you wish.

Tip:

If you like a bit of zip, add curry powder in place of paprika.

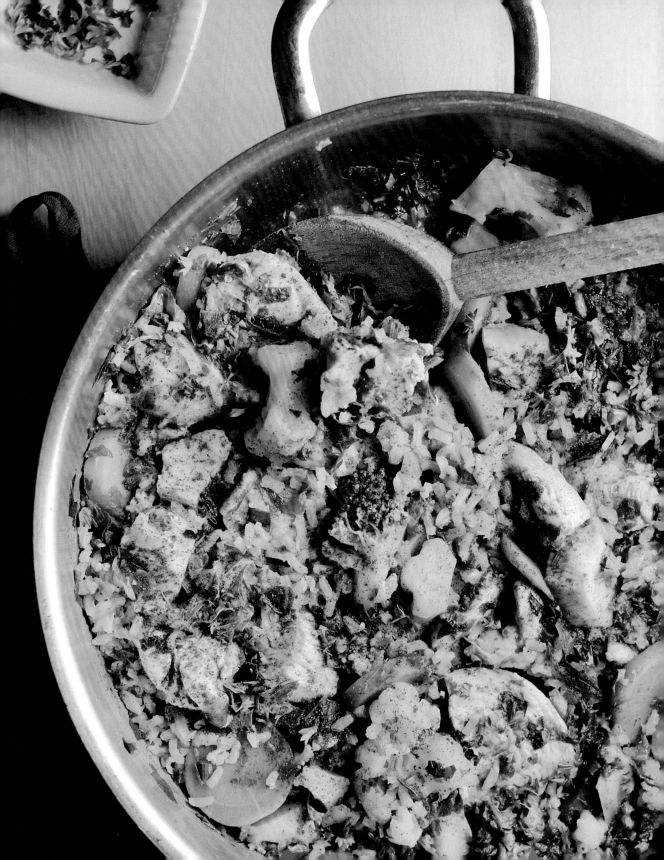

SLOW
COOKER

Slow-Cooker Chicken and Salsa

Marcia S. Myer, Manheim, PA

Makes 6 servings

Prep. Time: 10 minutes   Cooking Time: 4–10 hours   Ideal slow-cooker size: 5-qt.

2 (15-oz.) cans black beans

1½ lb. boneless chicken breasts, cut into serving-size pieces

16-oz. jar black bean salsa

16-oz. jar corn salsa

1 cup uncooked brown rice

2 cups water

1 cup sour cream

1 cup shredded cheddar cheese or Mexican blend cheese

1 avocado, sliced, for garnish

Corn chips, for garnish

1. Combine the beans, chicken, black bean salsa, corn salsa, brown rice, and 2 cups water in slow cooker.

2. Cook on High for 4 hours or on Low for 8–10 hours, adding water if needed near the end of the cooking time.

3. To serve, place 1½ cups of the chicken mixture on individual serving plates. Top with the sour cream and cheese. Garnish with the avocado and corn chips.

Tex-Mex Chicken Casserole

Ruth C. Hancock, Earlsboro, OK

Makes 6 servings

Prep. Time: 45 minutes ☙ Baking Time: 35 minutes

2 cups shredded rotisserie chicken meat

2 cups crushed tortilla chips

15-oz. can beans, rinsed and drained

1 cup corn kernels

⅔ cup sour cream

½–1 tsp. chili powder, according to your taste preference

2 cups salsa, *divided*

1 cup shredded cheese, *divided*

1. Combine chicken, chips, beans, corn, sour cream, and chili powder in mixing bowl.

2. Grease 2-quart baking dish.

3. Layer half of chicken mixture into baking dish.

4. Top with half of salsa.

5. Top with half of cheese.

6. Repeat steps 3–5.

7. Cover with foil.

8. Bake at 350°F for 25 minutes.

9. Uncover and bake 10 minutes more.

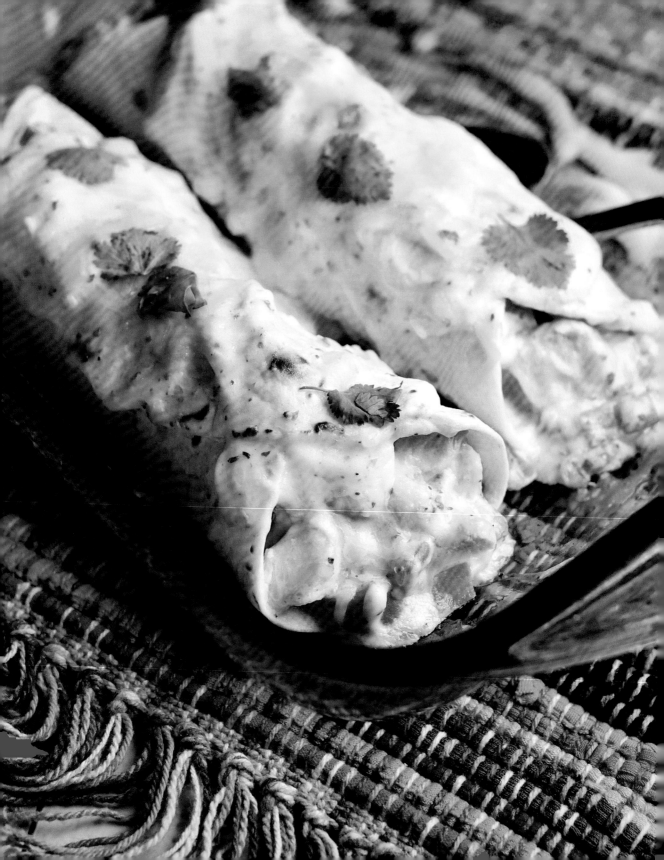

Creamy Chicken Enchilada

OVEN

Cheryl Martin, Turin, NY

Makes 10 servings

Prep. Time: 30 minutes   Baking Time: 30–40 minutes

2 (10¾-oz.) cans cream of chicken soup

8 oz. sour cream

¼ tsp. cumin

¼ tsp. oregano

3 cups diced, cooked chicken

4-oz. can chopped green chiles

1 tsp. chili powder

2 cups shredded cheddar cheese, *divided*

10 flour tortillas

1. In large mixing bowl, combine soup with sour cream, cumin, and oregano to make sauce.

2. In another bowl combine 1 cup sauce with chicken, green chiles, chili powder, and 1 cup shredded cheese.

3. Fill each soft tortilla with equal portion of chicken mixture.

4. Grease 9 × 13-inch glass baking dish.

5. Roll up tortillas. Arrange in baking dish.

6. Spoon remaining sauce over tortillas.

7. Sprinkle with remaining cheese.

8. Bake at 350°F for 30–40 minutes, or until enchiladas are heated through and sauce is bubbly.

Tips:

- You can make this ahead, and then refrigerate or freeze it until ready to bake! If frozen, thaw before baking.

- Barbecued chicken adds a tasty, bacon-like flavor to the dish.

- I like to use an ice cream scoop to divide the filling mixture equally between the tortillas.

SLOW COOKER

Cheesy Stuffed Peppers

Jean Moore, Pendleton, IN

Makes 8 servings

Prep. Time: 40 minutes ❧ Cooking Time: 3–9 hours
Ideal slow-cooker size: 6-qt. (or large enough so that all peppers sit on the bottom of the cooker)

8 small green bell peppers, tops removed and seeded

10-oz. pkg. frozen corn

¾ lb. lean ground turkey

¾ lb. extra-lean ground beef

8-oz. can tomato sauce

½ tsp. garlic powder

¼ tsp. black pepper

1 cup shredded cheddar cheese

½ tsp. Worcestershire sauce

¼ cup chopped onions

3 Tbsp. water

2 Tbsp. ketchup

1. Wash peppers and drain well. Combine all other ingredients except water and ketchup in mixing bowl. Stir well.

2. Stuff peppers ⅔ full of ground meat mixture.

3. Pour water in slow cooker. Arrange peppers on top.

4. Pour ketchup over peppers.

5. Cover. Cook on High for 3–4 hours or on Low for 7–9 hours.

Chicken Rice Bake

Nanci Keatley, Salem, OR

Makes 6 servings

Prep. Time: 20 minutes   ❧   Baking Time: 1½ hours   ❧   Standing Time: 10 minutes

2 lb. boneless skinless chicken breasts, cut into bite-sized pieces

3½ cups low-sodium chicken broth

1½ cups uncooked brown rice

1 cup chopped celery

1 cup chopped carrots

1 cup finely diced onions

2 cups sliced fresh mushrooms

1½ tsp. salt

1 tsp. pepper

1 tsp. dill weed

1 tsp. garlic, chopped

1. Spray a 2-quart baking dish with nonstick cooking spray.

2. Combine all ingredients in large mixing bowl.

3. Spoon into baking dish. Bake at 350°F for 1½ hours.

4. Allow to stand 10 minutes before serving.

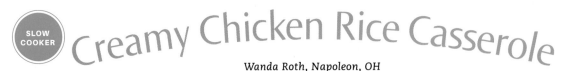

Creamy Chicken Rice Casserole

Wanda Roth, Napoleon, OH

Makes 8 servings

Prep. Time: 20 minutes ♣ Cooking Time: 2–6 hours ♣ Ideal slow-cooker size: 6-qt.

1 cup long-grain rice, uncooked

3 cups water

2 tsp. low-sodium chicken bouillon granules

10¾-oz. can cream of chicken soup

2 cups chopped, cooked chicken breast

¼ tsp. garlic powder

1 tsp. onion salt

1 cup grated cheddar cheese

16-oz. bag frozen broccoli, thawed

1. Combine all ingredients except broccoli in slow cooker.

2. Cook on High for 2–3 hours or on Low for 4–6 hours.

3. One hour before end of cooking time, stir in broccoli.

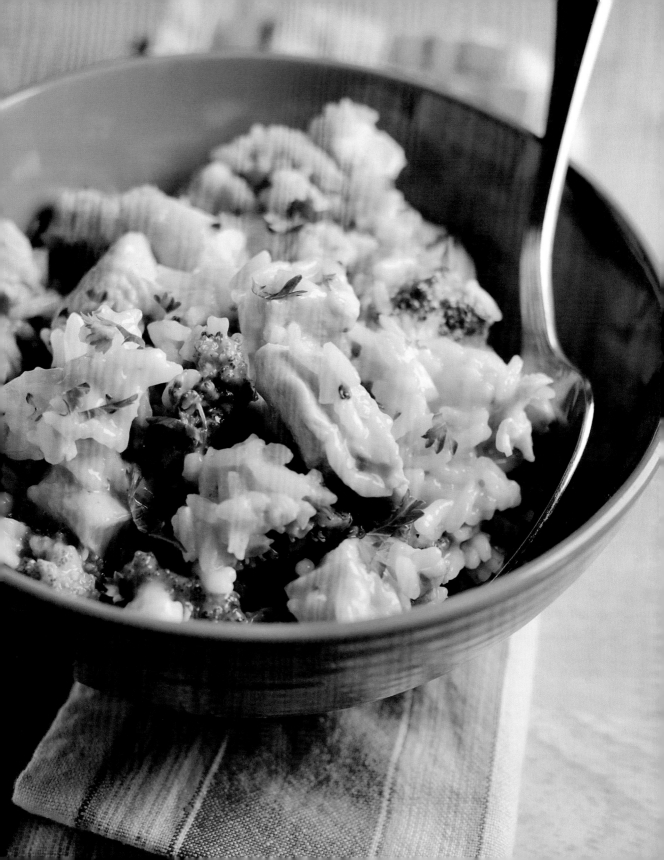

Maple-Glazed Turkey Breast with Rice

Jeanette Oberholtzer, Manheim, PA

Makes 4 servings

Prep. Time: 10–15 minutes & *Cooking Time: 4–6 hours* & *Ideal slow-cooker size: 3- to 4-qt.*

6-oz. pkg. long-grain wild rice mix

1½ cups water

2-lb. boneless turkey breast, cut into 1½–2-inch chunks

¼ cup maple syrup

1 onion, chopped

¼ tsp. ground cinnamon

½ tsp. salt, *optional*

1. Combine all ingredients in slow cooker.

2. Cook on Low for 4–6 hours, or until turkey and rice are both tender, but not dry or mushy.

Chicken Bulgur Skillet

Alice Rush, Quakertown, PA

Makes 6 servings

Prep. Time: 15–20 minutes   *Cooking Time: 27–30 minutes*

I lb. boneless skinless chicken breast, cut into 1-inch cubes

2 tsp. olive oil

2 medium carrots, chopped

⅔ cup chopped onions

3 Tbsp. chopped walnuts

½ tsp. caraway seeds

¼ tsp. ground cumin

1½ cups uncooked bulgur

2 cups low-sodium chicken broth

2 Tbsp. raisins or dried cranberries

¼ tsp. salt

⅛ tsp. ground cinnamon

1. In large non-stick skillet, cook chicken in oil over medium-high heat until no longer pink. Remove chicken from skillet and keep warm.

2. In same skillet, stir-fry carrots, onions, nuts, caraway seeds, and cumin for 3–4 minutes, or until onion starts to brown.

3. Stir in bulgur. Gradually add broth.

4. Bring to a boil over medium-high heat. Reduce heat.

5. Add raisins or dried cranberries, salt, cinnamon, and chicken.

6. Cover and simmer 12–15 minutes, or until bulgur is tender.

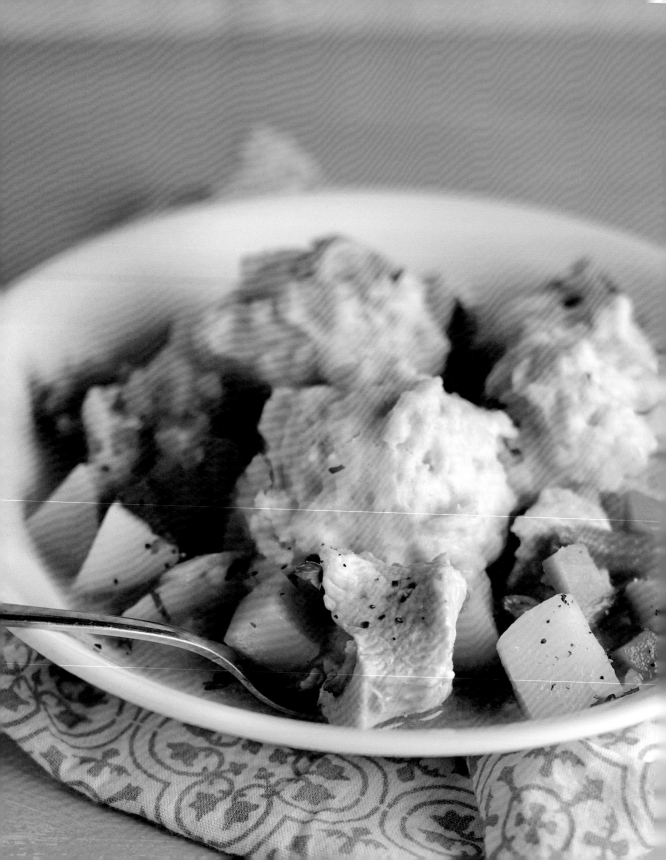

Chicken and Dumplings

Annabelle Unternahrer, Shipshewana, IN

Makes 5–6 servings

Prep. Time: 25 minutes 	 Cooking Time: 2½–3½ hours 	 Ideal slow-cooker size: 3- or 4-qt.

1 lb. uncooked boneless, skinless chicken breasts, cut in 1-inch cubes

1 lb. frozen vegetables of your choice

1 medium onion, diced

3 cups chicken broth, *divided*

1½ cups low-fat buttermilk biscuit mix

1. Combine chicken, vegetables, onion, and chicken broth (reserve ½ cup, plus 1 Tbsp., broth) in slow cooker.

2. Cover. Cook on High for 2–3 hours.

3. Mix biscuit mix with reserved broth until moistened. Drop by tablespoonfuls over hot chicken and vegetables.

4. Cover. Cook on High for 10 minutes.

5. Uncover. Cook on High for 20 minutes more.

Wild 'N Tangy BBQ Chicken

Maria Shevlin, Sicklerville, NJ

Makes 4–6 servings

Prep. Time: 15 minutes ♣ Cooking Time: 15 minutes

1–2 lb. boneless, skinless chicken thighs

1–2 lb. boneless, skinless chicken breasts

1 cup chicken broth

1 tsp. onion powder

1 tsp. garlic powder

½–1 tsp. chili powder

¼–½ tsp. red pepper flakes

½ tsp. smoked paprika

¼ cup brown sugar

½ cup onion, minced

1½ tsp. parsley flakes

2 cloves garlic, minced

18-oz. bottle of your favorite barbecue sauce

1. Place all the ingredients, except the barbecue sauce, into the inner pot of the Instant Pot.

2. Secure the lid and set the vent to sealing. Manually set the cook time for 15 minutes on high pressure.

3. When cook time is up, let the pressure release naturally for 10 minutes, then manually release the remaining pressure.

4. When the pin drops, remove the lid. Carefully drain most of the broth out and reserve it.

5. Shred the chicken in the pot with your hand mixer or between 2 forks. Note: The hand mixer works like a charm!

6. Add the BBQ sauce and mix well.

7. Taste and adjust seasonings if needed. If it's too dry for your liking, add some of the reserved liquid.

Serving suggestion:

Either serve on a plate, or on slider buns with a side of coleslaw and pickles. You can also try serving it open-faced on Texas toast.

Pork

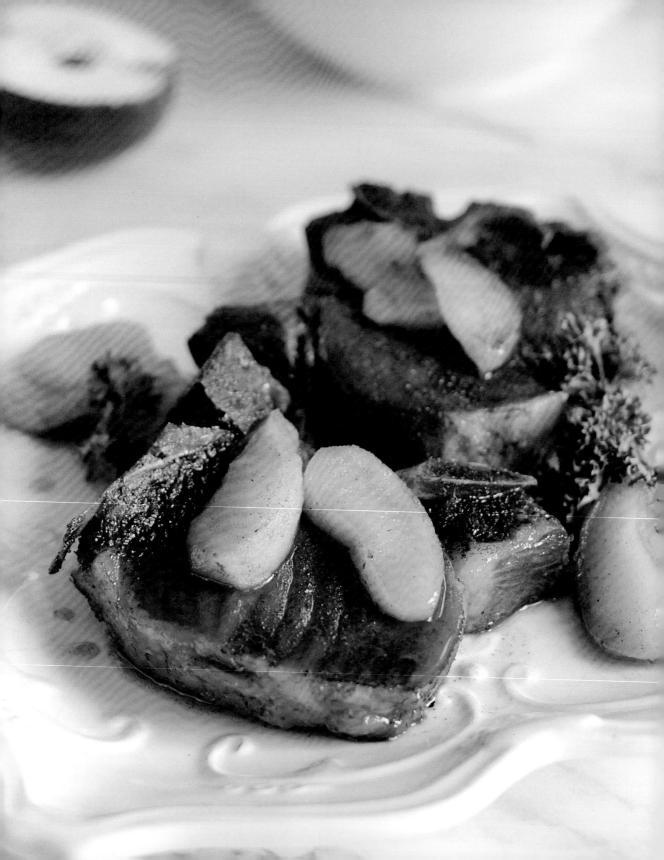

Pork Chops with Apple Pie Filling and Stuffing

Arlene M. Kopp, Lineboro, MD

Makes 6 servings

Prep. Time: 15 minutes ⚬ Cooking Time: 2–3 hours ⚬ Ideal slow-cooker size: oval 6- or 7-qt.

4 large baking apples, cored and sliced, peeled or unpeeled

¼ cup brown sugar

1 tsp. cinnamon

Salt and pepper to taste

6 (¾-inch-thick) bone-in, blade-cut pork chops

1. Grease the interior of a slow-cooker crock.

2. Scatter the apple slices over bottom of crock.

3. Sprinkle with the brown sugar and cinnamon.

4. Salt and pepper each chop on both sides. Place on top of the apples.

5. Cover. Cook on Low for 2–3 hours, or until an instant-read thermometer registers 140°F–145°F.

6. Serve on a platter, topped with apples.

SLOW COOKER

Applesauce Pork Chops with Sweet Potatoes

Hope Comerford, Clinton Township, MI

Makes 4 servings

Prep. Time: 5 minutes ⚬ Cooking Time: 6 hours ⚬ Ideal slow-cooker size: 4-qt.

2 lb. thick-cut, bone-in pork chops

3 medium sweet potatoes, cut in 1-inch cubes

1½ cups natural applesauce

¼ cup brown sugar

1–2 Tbsp. minced onion

1 tsp. salt

¼ tsp. pepper

1. Place pork chops and sweet potatoes in crock.

2. In a bowl, mix the remaining ingredients. Pour this over the pork chops.

3. Cover and cook on Low for 6 hours.

Paprika Pork Chops with Rice

Sharon Easter, Yuba City, CA

Makes 4 servings

Prep. Time: 5 minutes   *Cooking Time: 30 minutes*

⅛ tsp. pepper

1 tsp. paprika

4–5 thick-cut, boneless pork chops (1–1½ inches thick)

1 Tbsp. olive oil

1¼ cups water, *divided*

1 onion, sliced

½ green bell pepper, sliced in rings

1½ cups canned no-salt-added stewed tomatoes

1 cup brown rice

1. Mix the pepper and paprika in a flat dish. Dredge the chops in the seasoning mixture.

2. Set the Instant Pot to the Sauté function and heat the oil in the inner pot.

3. Brown the chops on both sides for 1–2 minutes a side. Remove the pork chops and set aside.

4. Pour a small amount of water into the inner pot and scrape up any bits from the bottom with a wooden spoon. Press Cancel.

5. Place the browned chops side by side in the inner pot. Place 1 slice onion and 1 ring of green pepper on top of each chop. Spoon tomatoes with their juices over the top.

6. Pour the rice in and pour the remaining water over the top.

7. Secure the lid and set the vent to sealing.

8. Manually set the cook time for 30 minutes on high pressure.

9. When the cooking time is over, manually release the pressure.

INSTANT POT

Pork Chops with Potatoes and Green Beans

Hope Comerford, Clinton Township, MI

Makes 4 servings

Prep. Time: 8 minutes   *Cooking Time: 13 minutes*

2 Tbsp. olive oil, *divided*

4 boneless pork chops, 1–1½ inches thick

Salt and pepper to taste

1 cup chicken broth

2 lb. baby potatoes, sliced in half

1 lb. fresh green beans, ends trimmed

3 cloves garlic, crushed

2 tsp. salt

1 tsp. onion powder

1 tsp. dried rosemary

½ tsp. dried thyme

¼ tsp. pepper

1. Set the Instant Pot to Sauté and let it get hot. Add 1 tablespoon of the oil.

2. Sprinkle each side of the pork chops with salt and pepper. Brown them on each side in the Instant Pot. Remove them when done.

3. Pour in the broth and scrape the bottom of the pot, bringing up any stuck-on bits. Press Cancel.

4. Arrange the pork chops back in the inner pot of the Instant Pot.

5. In a medium bowl, toss the potatoes and green beans with the garlic, salt, onion powder, rosemary, thyme, and pepper. Pour them over the pork chops.

6. Secure the lid and set the vent to sealing. Manually set the cook time for 8 minutes on high pressure.

7. When cook time is up, let the pressure release naturally for 10 minutes, then manually release the remaining pressure.

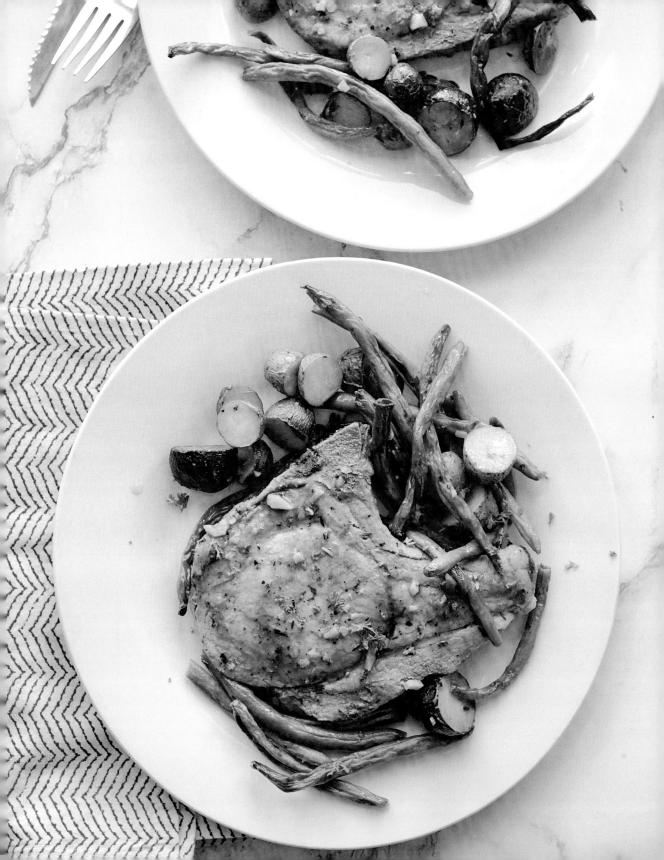

Tropical Pork with Yams

Hope Comerford, Clinton Township, MI

Makes 6 servings

Prep. Time: 15 minutes ⚬ *Cooking Time: 7–8 hours* ⚬ *Ideal slow-cooker size: 5-qt.*

2–3-lb. pork loin

Salt and pepper to taste

20-oz. can crushed pineapple

¼ cup honey

¼ cup brown sugar

¼ cup apple cider vinegar

1 tsp. low-sodium soy sauce

4 yams, cut into bite-sized chunks

1. Spray the crock with nonstick spray.

2. Lay the pork loin at the bottom of the crock and sprinkle it with salt and pepper on both sides.

3. In a separate bowl, combine the pineapple, honey, brown sugar, apple cider vinegar, and soy sauce. Mix well.

4. Place the chunks of yams over and around the pork loin and then pour the pineapple sauce over the top.

5. Cover and cook on Low for 7–8 hours.

Cranberry Jalapeño Pork Roast

Hope Comerford, Clinton Township, MI

Makes 4–6 servings

Prep. Time: 10 minutes   *Cooking Time: 7–8 hours*   *Ideal slow-cooker size: 3-qt.*

2–3-lb. pork roast

3 medium potatoes, cut in 1-inch chunks

1 tsp. garlic powder

½ tsp. salt

½ tsp. pepper

1 small onion, chopped

½ jalapeño, seeded and diced

14-oz. can jellied cranberry sauce

1. Place pork roast and potatoes in crock.

2. Season with the garlic powder, salt, and pepper.

3. Dump in the onion and jalapeño.

4. Spoon the jellied cranberry sauce over the top of the contents of the crock.

5. Cover and cook on Low for 7–8 hours.

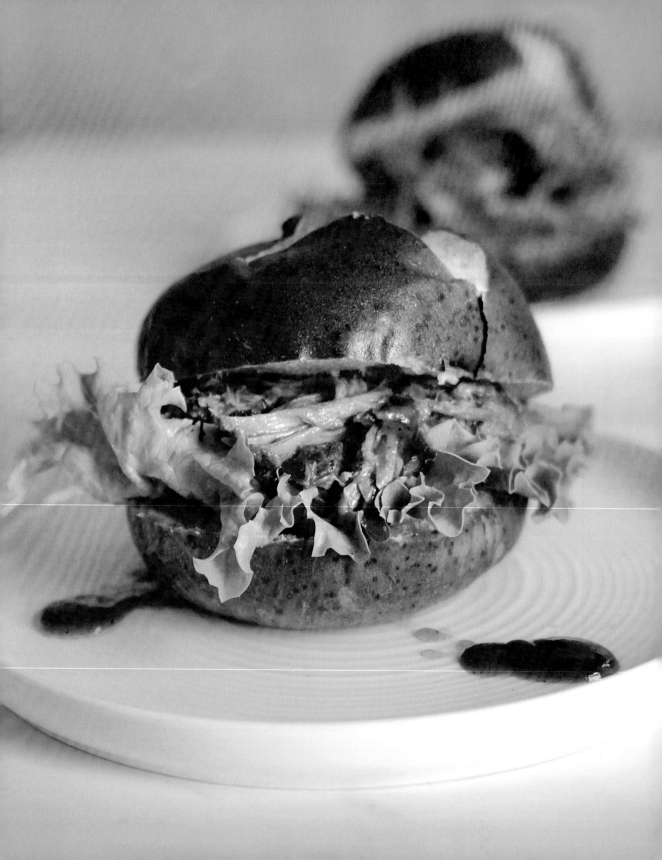

BBQ Pork Sandwiches

INSTANT POT

Carol Eveleth, Cheyenne, WY

Makes 4 servings

Prep. Time: 20 minutes ⚬ Cooking Time: 60 minutes

2 tsp. salt

I tsp. onion powder

I tsp. garlic powder

I Tbsp. olive oil

2-lb. pork shoulder roast, cut into 3-inch pieces

2 cups barbecue sauce

1. In a small bowl, combine the salt, onion powder, and garlic powder. Season the pork with the rub.

2. Turn the Instant Pot on to Sauté. Heat the olive oil in the inner pot.

3. Add the pork to the oil and turn to coat. Lock the lid and set vent to sealing.

4. Press Manual and cook on high pressure for 45 minutes.

5. When cooking is complete, release the pressure manually, then open the lid.

6. Using 2 forks, shred the pork, pour barbecue sauce over the pork, then press Sauté. Simmer 3–5 minutes. Press Cancel. Toss pork to mix.

Serving suggestion:

Pile the shredded BBQ pork on the bottom half of a bun. Add any additional toppings if you wish, then finish with the top half of the bun.

Italian Sausage and Potatoes

Maryann Markano, Wilmington, DE

Makes 4 servings

Prep. Time: 20 minutes   Roasting Time: 30–35 minutes

I lb. sweet or hot Italian sausage, cut on the diagonal in 1½-inch lengths

I lb. small red potatoes, each cut in half

I large onion, cut into 12 wedges

2 red or yellow bell peppers, cut into strips

I Tbsp. olive oil

1. Preheat the oven to 450°F.

2. In a large bowl or a plastic bag, combine all the ingredients. Toss to coat the meat and vegetables with oil.

3. Pour the mixture onto a large, lightly greased jelly-roll pan.

4. Roast for 30–35 minutes, or until the potatoes are fork-tender and the sausages are lightly browned. Stir halfway through cooking.

Smoked Sausage and Sauerkraut

Joan Terwilliger, Lebanon, PA

Makes 6–8 servings

Prep. Time: 20 minutes   ⚬   Baking Time: 1¾–2 hours

2 Tbsp. butter

3 apples, peeled, halved, sliced thickly

1 large sweet onion, halved, sliced thickly

4 Yukon Gold potatoes, peeled, cut in ½-inch cubes

½ cup light brown sugar, packed

¼ cup Dijon mustard

½–1 lb. kielbasa, sliced ½-inch thick, depending on amount of meat you like

1 cup apple cider, or Riesling

2 lb. sauerkraut, rinsed and drained

1. Melt butter in large oven-proof Dutch oven over medium-high heat.

2. Sauté apples and onion 10 minutes in butter, stirring occasionally.

3. Add potatoes.

4. In small bowl, mix the sugar and mustard. Add to onion-potato mixture.

5. Place sausage slices on top of onion-potato mixture.

6. Pour in cider or wine.

7. Place sauerkraut on top of sausage.

8. Bake, covered, at 350°F for 1¾–2 hours, or until potatoes are tender.

Carnitas

Hope Comerford, Clinton Township, MI

Makes 12 servings

Prep. Time: 10 minutes ❧ Cooking Time: 10–12 hours ❧ Ideal slow-cooker size: 4-qt.

2-lb. pork shoulder roast

1½ tsp. kosher salt

½ tsp. pepper

2 tsp. cumin

5 cloves garlic, minced

1 tsp. oregano

3 bay leaves

2 cups low-sodium chicken stock

2 Tbsp. lime juice

1 tsp. lime zest

Corn tortillas

1. Place the pork shoulder roast in the slow cooker crock.

2. In a bowl, mix the salt, pepper, cumin, garlic, and oregano. Rub the mixture onto the pork roast.

3. Place the bay leaves around the pork roast, then pour in the chicken stock around the roast, being careful not to wash off the spices.

4. Cover and cook on Low for 10–12 hours.

5. Remove the roast with a slotted spoon, as well as the bay leaves. Shred the pork between two forks, then replace the shredded pork in the crock and stir.

6. Add the lime juice and lime zest to the crock and stir.

7. Serve on warmed white corn tortillas.

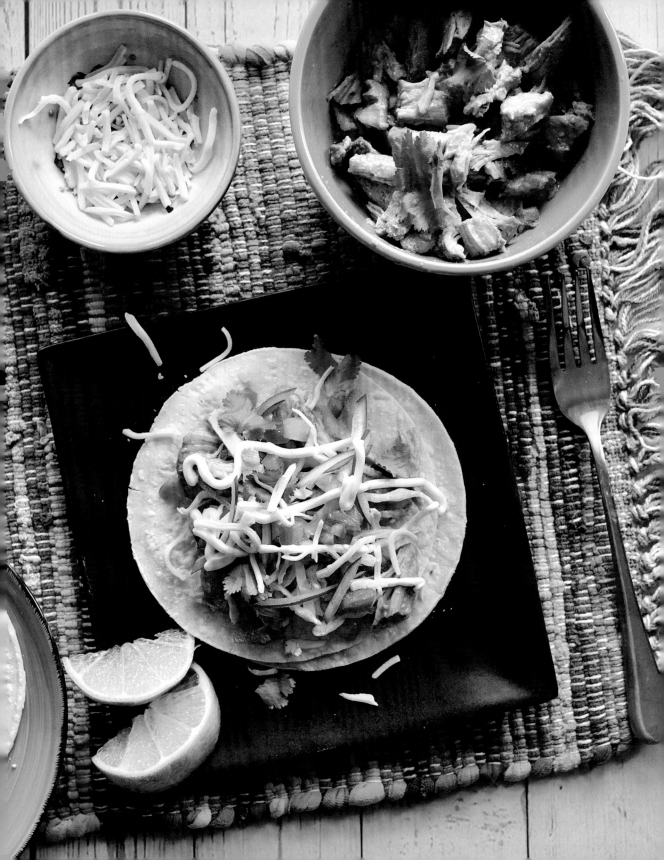

INSTANT POT

Rice with Beans and Franks

Maria Shevlin, Sicklerville, NJ

Makes 4–6 servings

Prep. Time: 8 minutes ⚬ *Cooking Time: 10 minutes*

1 tsp. olive oil

1 sweet onion, diced

4–6 slices bacon, uncooked, sliced

¾ cup ketchup

2 Tbsp. yellow mustard (you can also use Dijon for a slight kick)

2 tsp. Worcestershire sauce

1 Tbsp. parsley flakes

1 tsp. garlic powder

1 tsp. onion powder

½–1 tsp. chili powder

¼ tsp. red pepper flakes

3 (15-oz.) cans of your favorite baked beans (we enjoy a variety of Bush's)

8 hot dogs, any type, sliced into rounds

1–2 cups precooked rice, for serving

1. Set the Instant Pot to Sauté and heat up the olive oil. Add the diced onion and bacon. Cook until onions soften and bacon is almost cooked through, not crisp.

2. Add the ketchup, mustard, Worcestershire sauce, parsley flakes, garlic powder, onion powder, chili powder, and red pepper flakes. Stir.

3. Add in the beans, then hot dogs. Mix all together one final time.

4. Place the lid on and let it cook for 10 minutes.

5. When the 10 minutes is up, remove the lid and stir in the cooked rice. Press Cancel.

Serving suggestion:

Serve with a side salad and buttered rolls. Top with sliced scallions or more diced sweet onion.

Stromboli

Monica Leaman Kehr, Portland, MI

Makes 6 servings

Prep. Time: 20 minutes   Rising Time: 30–40 minutes
Baking Time: 20 minutes   Standing Time: 10 minutes

1 loaf frozen bread dough, thawed
(see package directions)

Italian seasoning

2 cups grated mozzarella cheese

3 oz. sliced pepperoni

4 oz. chipped cooked ham

½ cup sliced black olives

⅓ cup sliced mushrooms, *optional*

2 Tbsp. chopped onions, *optional*

2 Tbsp. chopped green or red bell
pepper, *optional*

1. Roll thawed bread dough to 10 × 15-inch rectangle on lightly floured surface.

2. Sprinkle dough with Italian seasoning. Cover entire rectangle with cheese, pepperoni, ham, black olives, and any of the other ingredients you want. Press toppings down gently into dough.

3. Starting with the long side of the rectangle, roll dough up into a log shape. Seal ends by pinching dough together.

4. Carefully lift onto a lightly greased baking sheet. Cover and allow to rise 30–40 minutes.

5. Bake on sheet for 20 minutes at 400°F, or until lightly browned.

6. Allow to stand for 10 minutes before slicing.

 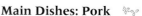

Cordon Bleu Stromboli

Melody Baum, Greencastle, PA

Makes 6 servings

Prep. Time: 15 minutes & Rising Time: 20 minutes
Baking Time: 25–30 minutes & Standing Time: 10 minutes

1 loaf frozen bread dough, thawed
(see package directions)

2 Tbsp. butter

8 oz. thinly sliced deli ham

½ cup shredded Swiss cheese

5 oz. thinly sliced deli turkey

1. Roll the bread dough into an 8 × 10-inch rectangle on a baking sheet.

2. Spread with the butter. Top with a layer of ham, followed by a layer of cheese, and finally a layer of turkey.

3. Roll up, jelly-roll style, starting with the long side. Pinch the seam to seal and tuck the ends under.

4. Place seam-side down on a greased baking sheet. Set in a warm place. Cover with a tea towel and let rise for 20 minutes.

5. Bake at 350°F for 25–30 minutes, or until golden brown.

6. Allow to stand for 10 minutes before slicing.

Beef

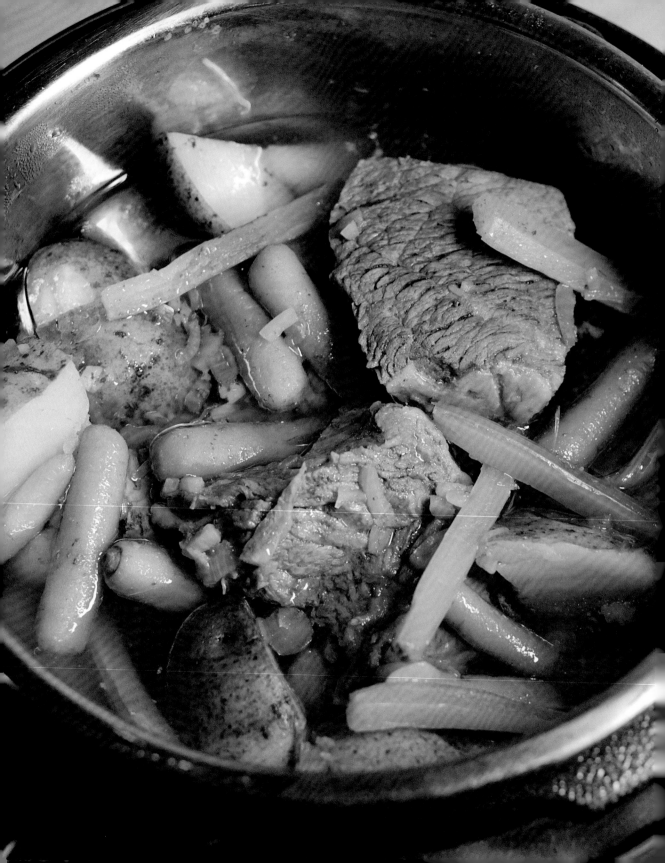

Easy Chuck Roast and Vegetables

INSTANT POT

Tina Houk, Clinton, MO
Arlene Wines, Newton, KS

Makes 6 servings

Prep. Time: 20 minutes ⚬ Cooking Time: 35 minutes

3–4 lb. chuck roast, trimmed of fat and cut into serving-sized chunks

4 medium potatoes, cubed, unpeeled

4 medium carrots, sliced, or 1 lb. baby carrots

2 celery ribs, sliced thin

1 pkg. dry onion soup mix

3 cups water

1. In an Instant Pot, combine the chuck roast chunks with the potatoes, carrots, and celery.

2. Mix together the onion soup mix and water and pour over the contents of the Instant Pot.

3. Secure the lid and make sure the vent is set to sealing. Set the Instant Pot to Manual mode for 35 minutes on high pressure.

4. Let the pressure release naturally when the cook time is up.

INSTANT POT

Pot Roast

Carole Whaling, New Tripoli, PA

Makes 8 servings

Prep. Time: 20 minutes   *Cooking Time: 35 minutes*

2 Tbsp. olive oil

3–4-lb. rump roast, or pot roast,
bone removed, and cut into
serving-sized pieces, trimmed of fat

4 medium potatoes, cubed or sliced

4 medium carrots, sliced

1 medium onion, sliced

1 tsp. salt

½ tsp. pepper

1 cup low-sodium beef broth

1. Press the Sauté button on the Instant Pot and add the olive oil. Once the oil is heated, lightly brown the pieces of roast, about 2 minutes on each side. Press Cancel.

2. Leave roast in Instant Pot and add the veggies around the roast, along with the salt, pepper, and beef broth.

3. Secure the lid and make sure the vent is set to sealing. Set the Instant Pot to Manual mode for 35 minutes. Let pressure release naturally when cook time is up.

Ready-When-You-Get-Home-Dinner

Beatrice Orgish, Richardson, TX

Makes: 6 servings

Prep. Time: 10–15 minutes ⚜ *Cooking Time: 4–5 hours* ⚜ *Ideal slow-cooker size: 5-qt.*

1 cup uncooked wild rice, rinsed and drained

1 cup chopped celery

1 cup chopped carrots

2 (4-oz.) cans mushrooms, drained

1 large onion, chopped

1 clove garlic, minced

½ cup slivered almonds

3 beef bouillon cubes

2½ tsp. seasoned salt

2 lb. boneless beef chuck roast, cut into 1½-inch pieces

3 cups water

1. Grease interior of slow-cooker crock.

2. Place ingredients in order listed into slow-cooker.

3. Cover. Cook on Low 4–5 hours or until beef and rice are tender. Stir before serving.

Variation:

Add a bay leaf and 4–6 whole peppercorns to mixture before cooking. Remove before serving.

Barbecue Sloppy Joes

Winifred Paul, Scottdale, PA

Makes 5 sandwiches

Prep. Time: 10 minutes ❧ Cooking Time: 15 minutes

¾ lb. ground beef
1 Tbsp. oil
1 tsp. lemon juice
1 Tbsp. vinegar
2 Tbsp. water
½ cup ketchup
1 tsp. brown sugar
1 tsp. onion, chopped fine
⅓ cup chopped celery
1 tsp. mustard powder
5 burger buns

1. Brown beef in oil in skillet. Stir frequently to break up clumps and to make sure meat browns completely. Drain off drippings.

2. Make sauce by combining lemon juice, vinegar, water, ketchup, brown sugar, onion, celery, and mustard in saucepan.

3. Heat thoroughly, but do not cook enough to soften vegetables.

4. When beginning to simmer, combine with meat.

5. Serve on buns.

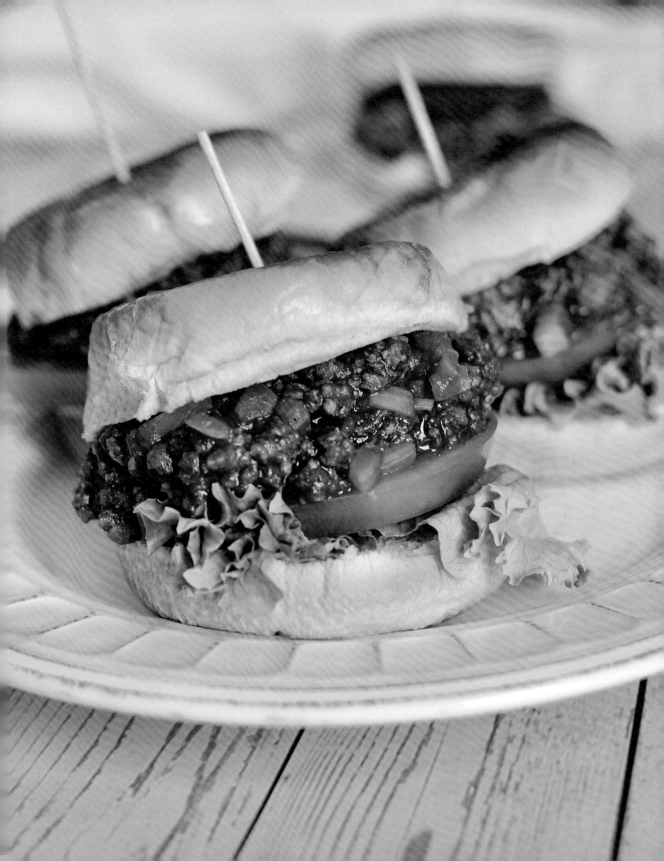

Hot Beef Sandwiches

Hope Comerford, Clinton Township, MI

Makes 12 servings

Prep. Time: 5 minutes & *Cooking Time: 60 minutes*

3-lb. rump roast

2 cups beef broth

2 (0.87-oz.) pkgs. beef gravy mix

1 tsp. garlic powder

1 tsp. onion powder

¼ tsp. pepper

6–8 slices of bread

1. Place the roast into the inner pot of the Instant Pot.

2. Mix the beef broth with beef gravy mix, garlic powder, onion powder, and pepper. Pour it over the roast.

3. Secure the lid and set the vent to sealing. Manually set the cook time for 60 minutes on high pressure.

4. When the cook time is over, let the pressure release naturally.

5. When the pin drops, remove the lid. Remove the beef to a bowl and shred it between two forks. Stir it back through the sauce in the inner pot.

6. Serve over slices of bread.

Steak and Rice Dinner

Susan Scheel, West Fargo, ND

Makes 8 servings

Prep. Time: 15–20 minutes ⚹ *Cooking Time: 4–6 hours* ⚹ *Ideal slow-cooker size: 5-qt.*

1 cup uncooked wild rice,
rinsed and drained

1 cup chopped celery

1 cup chopped carrots

2 (4-oz.) cans mushrooms, drained

1 large onion, chopped

½ cup slivered almonds

3 beef bouillon cubes

2½ tsp. seasoned salt

2 lb. boneless round steak,
cut in bite-sized pieces

3 cups water

1. Layer ingredients in slow cooker in order listed. Do not stir.

2. Cover. Cook on Low for 4–6 hours.

3. Stir before serving.

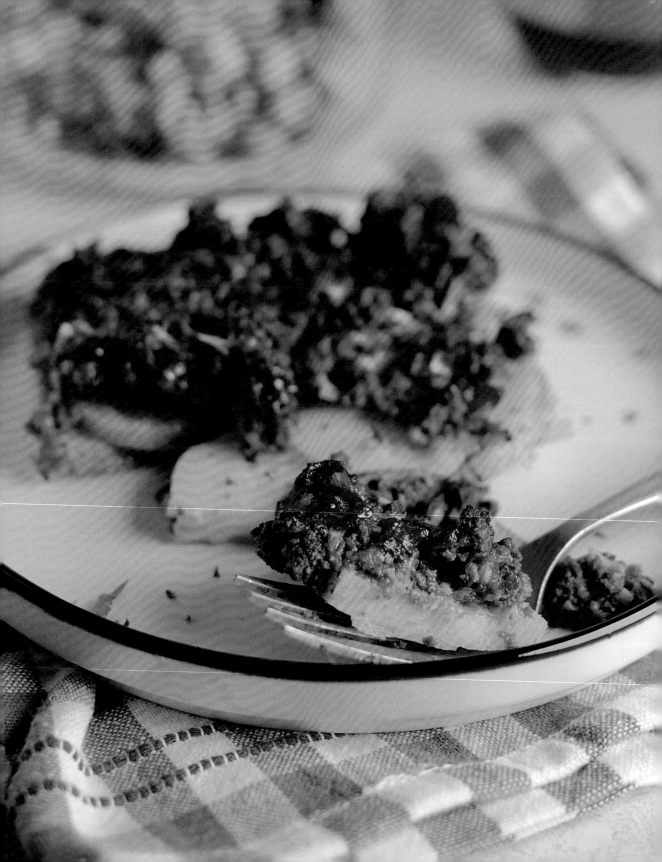

Beef and Potato Loaf

Deb Martin, Gap, PA

Makes 4–5 servings

Prep. Time: 15 minutes ⚬ Baking Time: 1 hour

4 cups raw, thinly sliced potatoes,
peeled or unpeeled

½ cup grated cheese

½ tsp. salt

¼ tsp. pepper

I lb. ground beef

¾ cup evaporated milk, or tomato juice

½ cup quick oats

½ cup chopped onion

Dash pepper

I tsp. seasoning salt

¼–½ cup ketchup

1. Arrange potatoes evenly over bottom of greased 9 × 13-inch baking pan.

2. Layer cheese across potatoes.

3. Sprinkle with ½ tsp. salt and ¼ tsp. pepper.

4. In a mixing bowl, mix the ground beef, evaporated milk or tomato juice, oats, onion, pepper, seasoning salt, and ketchup.

5. When well blended, crumble meat mixture evenly over potatoes and cheese.

6. Drizzle with ketchup.

7. Bake at 350°F for 1 hour, or until potatoes are tender. Check after 45 minutes of baking. If loaf is getting too dark, cover with foil for remainder of baking time.

Hearty Meat and Veggies Pilaf

Linda Yoder, Fresno, OH

Makes 6 servings

Prep. Time: 15 minutes   Cooking Time: 20 minutes

½ lb. ground beef, or venison

2 Tbsp. olive oil

1 cup sliced onions

1 clove garlic, minced

2 cups water

1 cup long-grain rice, uncooked

¼ lb. fresh mushrooms, sliced, or 4-oz. can sliced or cut-up mushrooms, drained

1 beef bouillon cube

1 tsp. salt

1 pint fresh green beans, or 1 lb. frozen green beans, thawed

½ tsp. basil

½ tsp. sage

½ tsp. oregano

½ tsp. marjoram

½ tsp. rosemary

½ tsp. thyme

¼ tsp. black pepper

1. In large nonstick skillet, brown ground beef in oil. Stir frequently to break up clumps, until no longer pink. Drain off any drippings.

2. Stir in onions and garlic, sautéing until tender.

3. Add water, cover, and bring to boil.

4. Stir in rice, mushrooms, bouillon, salt, green beans, basil, sage, oregano, marjoram, rosemary, thyme, and pepper.

5. Bring mixture again to boil, stirring once or twice.

6. Reduce heat, cover, and simmer 20 minutes, or until rice and green beans are tender.

7. Taste and correct seasoning if needed.

Tip:

If you prefer your green beans to have some crunch, add them to the skillet 10 minutes before the end of the cooking time.

Un-Stuffed Peppers

STOVETOP

Pat Bechtel, Dillsburg, PA
Sharon Miller, Holmesville, OH

Makes 6 servings

Prep. Time: 10–12 minutes ✿ *Cooking/Baking Time: 25 minutes*

1 lb. ground beef
10-oz. jar spaghetti sauce
2 Tbsp. barbecue sauce, *optional*
2 large green peppers (3–4 cups), coarsely chopped
1¼ cups water
1 cup instant rice

1. In a 12-inch nonstick skillet, brown the ground beef. Drain off the drippings.

2. Stir in all the remaining ingredients. Bring to a boil over high heat.

3. Reduce the heat to medium-low and cook, covered, for 20 minutes, or until the liquid is absorbed and the rice is tender.

Variation:

Instead of spaghetti sauce and water, substitute 4 cups tomato juice or V8 juice.

INSTANT POT

Walking Tacos

Hope Comerford, Clinton Township, MI

Makes 10–16 servings

Prep. Time: 10 minutes & Cooking Time: 15 minutes

2 lb. ground beef

2 tsp. garlic powder

2 tsp. onion powder

2 Tbsp. chili powder

I Tbsp. cumin

I Tbsp. onion powder

I Tbsp. garlic powder

I tsp. salt

½ tsp. oregano

½ tsp. red pepper flakes

I cup water

10–16 individual-sized bags of Doritos®

Suggested Toppings:

Diced tomatoes

Shredded cheese

Diced cucumbers

Chopped onion

Shredded lettuce

Sour cream

Salsa

1. Place the ground beef into the inner pot of the Instant Pot.

2. In a bowl, mix all the spices. Sprinkle over the beef. Pour the water around the beef.

3. Secure the lid and set the vent to sealing.

4. Manually set the cook time for 15 minutes on high pressure.

5. When cook time is up, manually release the pressure.

6. When the pin drops, remove the lid and break up the beef with a spoon.

7. To serve, open the bags of Doritos, crumble the chips in each bag with your hand, add some of the ground beef to the bag, then any additional toppings you desire. Serve each bag with a fork.

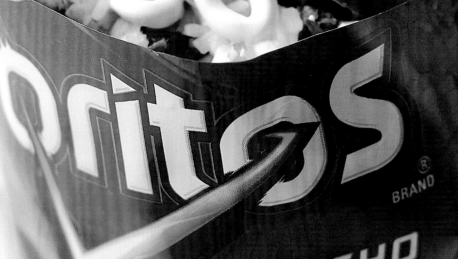

DUTCH
OVEN

Kodiak Casserole

Bev Beiler, Gap, PA

Makes 10 servings

Prep. Time: 15–25 minutes ⚖ *Baking Time: 60 minutes*

1 lb. ground beef

1–2 cups diced onions, depending on your taste preference

½ tsp. minced garlic

3 medium bell peppers, chopped

1 cup barbecue sauce

10¾-oz. can cream of tomato soup, undiluted

½ cup salsa

15-oz. can black beans, drained

4-oz. can mushroom stems and pieces, undrained

1 Tbsp. Worcestershire sauce

1 cup shredded cheddar cheese

1. In a Dutch oven, brown beef with onions and garlic. Stir frequently to break up meat, cooking until no pink remains. Drain off any drippings.

2. Stir peppers, barbecue sauce, soup, salsa, beans, mushrooms, and Worcestershire sauce into Dutch oven. Mix well.

3. Cover and bake at 350°F for 45 minutes.

4. Remove cover. Sprinkle with cheese. Continue baking 15 minutes, or until bubbly and heated through.

Reuben Casserole

Lois Ostrander, Lebanon, PA
Anne Townsend, Albuquerque, NM

Makes 6 servings

Prep. Time: 20–25 minutes   Baking Time: 45 minutes

16-oz. can sauerkraut, drained

12-oz. can corned beef, broken
into small pieces

3 cups shredded Swiss cheese

¼ cup mayonnaise

¼ cup Thousand Island dressing

2 medium tomatoes, sliced

4–5 cups rye or Italian bread, cubed

4 Tbsp. (½ stick) butter, melted

1. Spread sauerkraut over bottom of greased
9 × 9-inch baking dish.

2. Top with corned beef.

3. Sprinkle with shredded cheese.

4. In a small bowl, combine mayonnaise and
Thousand Island dressing. Spoon over cheese and
spread to cover.

5. Lay tomato slices over top of dressing.

6. Spread bread cubes over top of tomato slices.

7. Drizzle with melted butter.

8. Cover baking dish with foil. Bake at 350°F for
30 minutes.

9. Remove foil. Continue baking 15 more minutes.

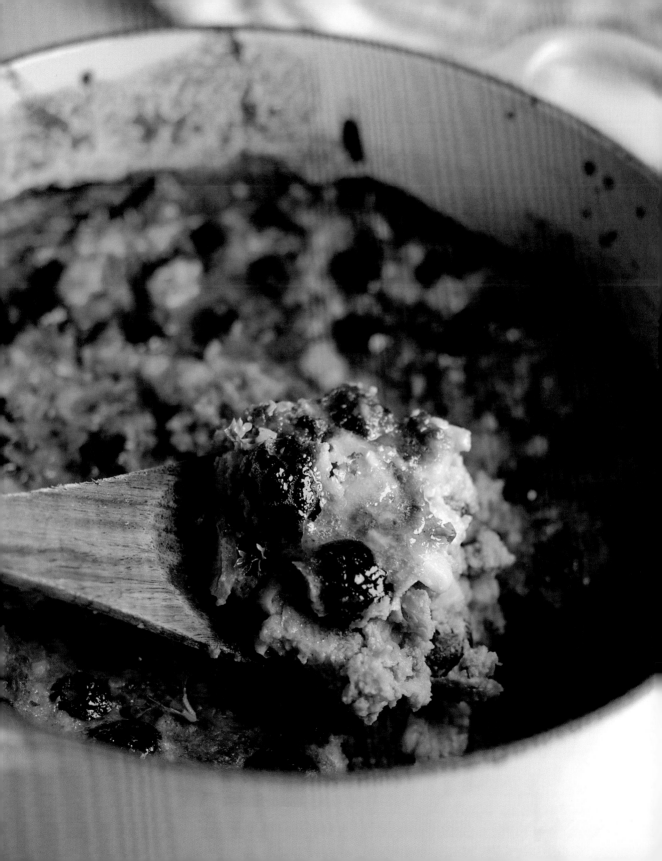

Tamale Pie

Joyce Bond, Stonyford, CA

Makes 8 servings

Prep. Time: 25 minutes ❧ Baking Time: 1 hour ❧ Standing Time: 5–10 minutes

1 Tbsp. olive oil
1 medium onion, chopped
2 lb. ground beef
1 clove garlic, minced
1 tsp. salt
½ tsp. pepper
3 Tbsp. chili powder
2 (8-oz.) cans tomato sauce
½ cup water
15-oz. can creamed corn
6-oz. can whole pitted olives, drained
1 cup evaporated milk
2 eggs, beaten
½ cup yellow cornmeal

1. Place olive oil and onion in 8-quart Dutch oven over medium heat. Cook, stirring frequently, until tender.

2. Add ground beef to onion in Dutch oven. Stir, breaking up clumps of meat, and cook until no longer pink. Drain off any drippings.

3. Off the stove, stir in garlic, salt, pepper, and chili powder.

4. Stir in tomato sauce and water.

5. Add creamed corn, olives, milk, eggs, and cornmeal. Mix well.

6. Place Dutch oven, uncovered, in oven at 375°F. Bake 1 hour until set.

7. Let stand 5–10 minutes before serving.

Meatless

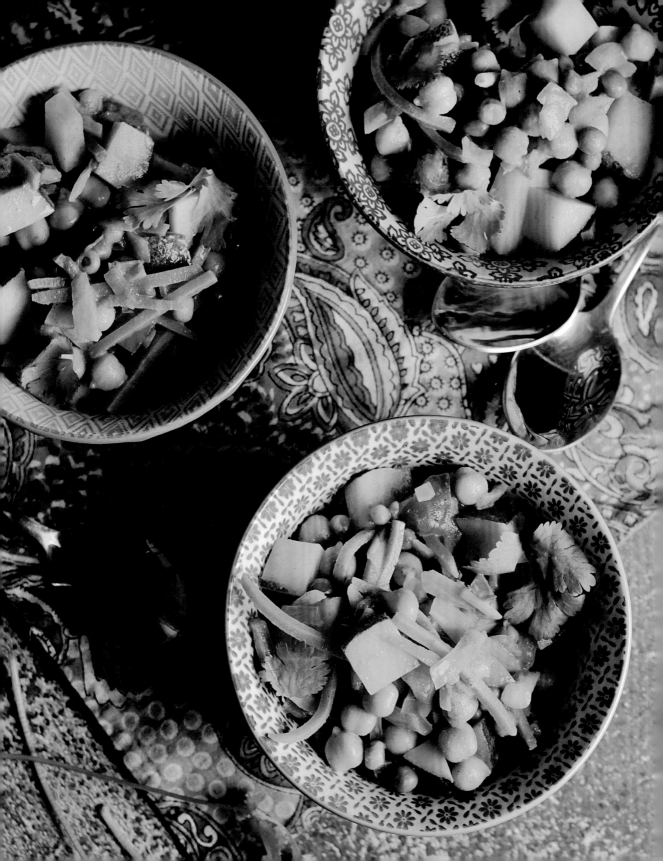

Thai Veggie Curry

Christen Chew, Lancaster, PA

Makes 4–5 servings

Prep. Time: 30 minutes ⚜ *Cooking Time: 5–6 hours* ⚜ *Ideal slow-cooker size: 4- or 5-qt.*

2 large carrots, thinly sliced

1 medium onion, chopped

3 cloves garlic, chopped

2 large potatoes, peeled or not, diced

15½-oz. can garbanzo beans, rinsed and drained

14½-oz. can diced tomatoes, undrained

2 Tbsp. curry powder

1 tsp. ground coriander

1 tsp. cayenne pepper

2 cups vegetable stock

½ cup frozen green peas

½ cup coconut milk

Salt to taste

1. Grease interior of slow-cooker crock.

2. Stir all ingredients except peas, coconut milk, and salt into crock. Mix well, making sure seasonings are distributed throughout.

3. Cover. Cook on Low for 5–6 hours, or until vegetables are as tender as you like them.

4. Just before serving, stir in peas and coconut milk. Season with salt to taste.

OVEN

Sun-Dried Tomato Casserole

Barbara Jean Fabel, Wausau, WI

Makes 12 servings

Prep. Time: 15–20 minutes ⚜ *Standing Time: 8 hours or overnight, plus 10 minutes* ⚜
Baking Time: 40 minutes

2 (9-oz.) pkgs. cheese ravioli
(look for them in the dairy case)

4 oz. sun-dried tomatoes in oil,
drained and chopped

1½ cups shredded cheddar cheese

1½ cups shredded Monterey
Jack cheese

8 eggs, beaten

2½ cups milk

1–2 Tbsp. fresh basil, snipped,
or 1–2 tsp. dried basil

1. Grease a 3-qt. baking dish. Place uncooked ravioli evenly in bottom.

2. Sprinkle ravioli with tomatoes. Top evenly with cheeses. Set aside.

3. In a mixing bowl, whisk eggs and milk until well combined. Pour over layers in casserole dish.

4. Cover and chill for 8 hours or overnight.

5. Bake, uncovered, at 350°F for 40 minutes, until center is set and knife inserted in center comes out clean.

6. Let stand 10 minutes before serving. Just before serving, sprinkle with basil.

Tip:

If you don't like sun-dried tomatoes, replace them with something you do like, such as sliced black olives or artichokes.

Chile Rellenos Casserole

OVEN

Elena Yoder, Albuquerque, NM

Makes 12 servings

Prep. Time: 30 minutes ⚬ *Baking Time: 35–40 minutes*

1 can (18–20) whole green chiles
1 lb. Monterey Jack cheese
Sprinkle garlic salt
4 eggs
1 Tbsp. flour
1 cup milk
¾ tsp. salt
¼–½ tsp. pepper
½ lb. cheddar, or longhorn, cheese, grated

1. Spray 9 × 13-inch baking pan with nonstick cooking spray.

2. Wearing gloves, cut chiles in half and remove seeds and membranes.

3. Cut Monterey Jack cheese into strips. Place strips in chili halves. Place stuffed chiles in pan side by side, cut side up.

4. Sprinkle with garlic salt.

5. In a mixing bowl, beat eggs. Stir in flour, milk, salt, and pepper.

6. Pour egg mixture over chiles.

7. Sprinkle with grated cheese.

8. Bake at 350°F for 35–40 minutes, or until set and beginning to brown.

Tip:

You can put this together the day before you want to serve it. Or stuff the chiles and freeze them until you need a quick meal. Then proceed with Step 5.

OVEN

Spicy Mexican Bean Burgers

Lois Hess, Lancaster, PA

Makes 4 burgers

Prep. Time: 30 minutes   Baking Time: 15–20 minutes

16-oz. can red kidney beans, rinsed, drained, and mashed

½ cup chopped onion

½ green bell pepper, chopped

1 carrot, steamed and mashed

⅛ cup salsa, your choice of flavors

1 cup whole wheat breadcrumbs

½ cup whole wheat flour

½ tsp. black pepper, *optional*

Dash chili powder

1. Preheat oven to 400°F.

2. Combine all ingredients in a good-sized bowl. Add more flour to create a firmer mixture or more salsa if mixture is too stiff.

3. Form into 4 balls and then flatten into patties.

4. Place on a baking sheet, lightly sprayed with cooking spray.

5. Bake 15–20 minutes, or until firm and brown.

Serving suggestion:

Serve on a whole wheat bun with lettuce, tomato, and salsa.

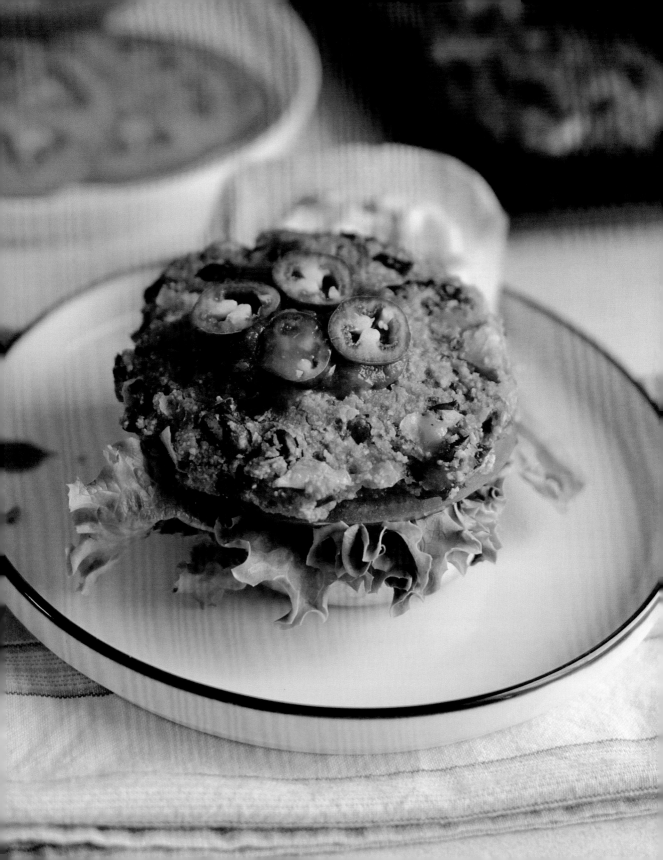

Seafood

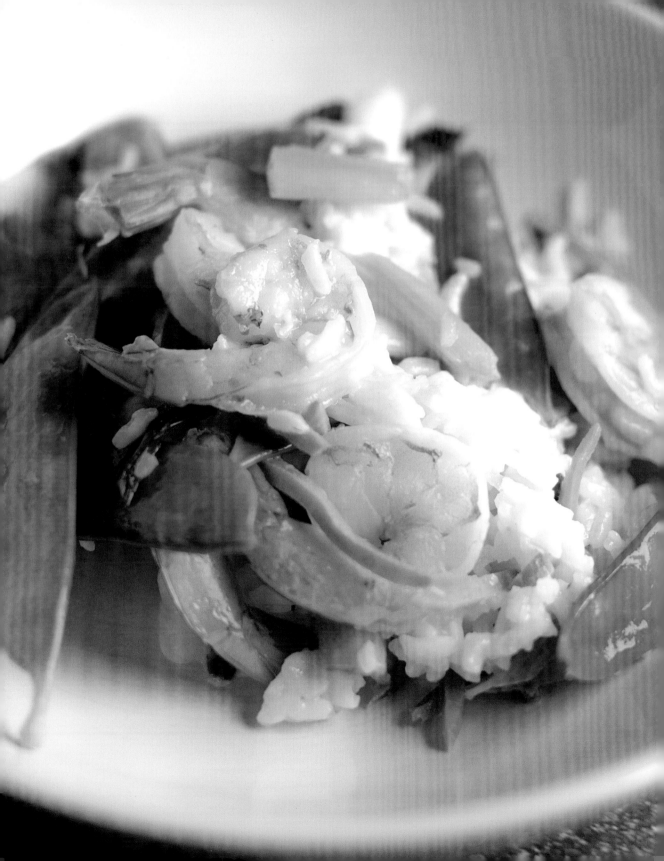

Thai Shrimp and Rice

Pat Bechtel, Dillsburg, PA

Makes 6 servings

Prep. Time: 10 minutes   Cooking Time: 25–30 minutes

1 tsp. olive oil

½ cup sliced scallions

1 Tbsp. chopped garlic

14-oz. can light coconut milk

1½ cups jasmine, or converted, white rice

1 cup shredded carrots

1 tsp. salt

12 oz. raw shrimp, peeled and deveined

2½ cups (about ½ lb.) fresh snow peas

2 tsp. lime zest

Lime wedges

Cilantro for garnish

1. Heat olive oil in a large skillet over medium heat. Sauté scallions and garlic.

2. Pour coconut milk into a quart measure. Add enough water to make 3¼ cups.

3. Add milk mixture to skillet and bring to a boil.

4. Stir in rice, carrots, and salt.

5. Cover. Reduce heat and simmer 12 minutes, or until rice is nearly tender.

6. Stir in shrimp, snow peas, and lime zest. If rice looks dry, add ¼ cup water.

7. Cover and bring to a simmer. Cook 3–4 minutes, or until shrimp and peas are crisp-tender.

8. Garnish with lime wedges and chopped cilantro just before serving.

OVEN

Salmon Loaf

Clara Yoder Byler, Hartville, OH

Makes 3–4 servings

Prep. Time: 15 minutes ❧ Baking Time: 1 hour ❧ Standing Time: 10 minutes

14¾-oz. can salmon, drained and flaked

½ cup mayonnaise

10¾-oz. can cream of celery soup

1 egg, beaten

1 cup dry breadcrumbs

½ cup chopped onion

1 Tbsp. lemon juice

1. Combine salmon, mayonnaise, soup, egg, breadcrumbs, onion, and lemon juice in a bowl.

2. Shape into loaf. Place in greased 8½ × 4½-inch loaf pan.

3. Bake at 350°F for 1 hour.

4. Allow to stand 10 minutes before slicing.

Flounder Zucchini Bundles

OVEN

Betty L. Moore, Plano, IL

Makes 4 servings

Prep. Time: 15 minutes ⚜ *Baking Time: 20 minutes*

4 (6-oz.) flounder fillets

¼ tsp. lemon pepper, *divided*

1 medium lemon, thinly sliced, *divided*

1 medium zucchini, cut into ¼-inch-thick slices, *divided*

12 cherry tomatoes, sliced, *divided*

¼ tsp. dill weed, *divided*

¼ tsp. dried basil, *divided*

1. Place 1 fillet on double thickness of 15 × 18-inch piece of heavy-duty foil.

2. Sprinkle with ¼ of lemon pepper.

3. Top with ¼ of lemon slices, zucchini, and tomatoes.

4. Sprinkle with ¼ of dill and basil.

5. Fold foil around fish and seal tightly. Place on baking sheet.

6. Repeat with other fillets.

7. Bake at 425°F for 15–20 minutes, or until fish flakes easily.

Pastas

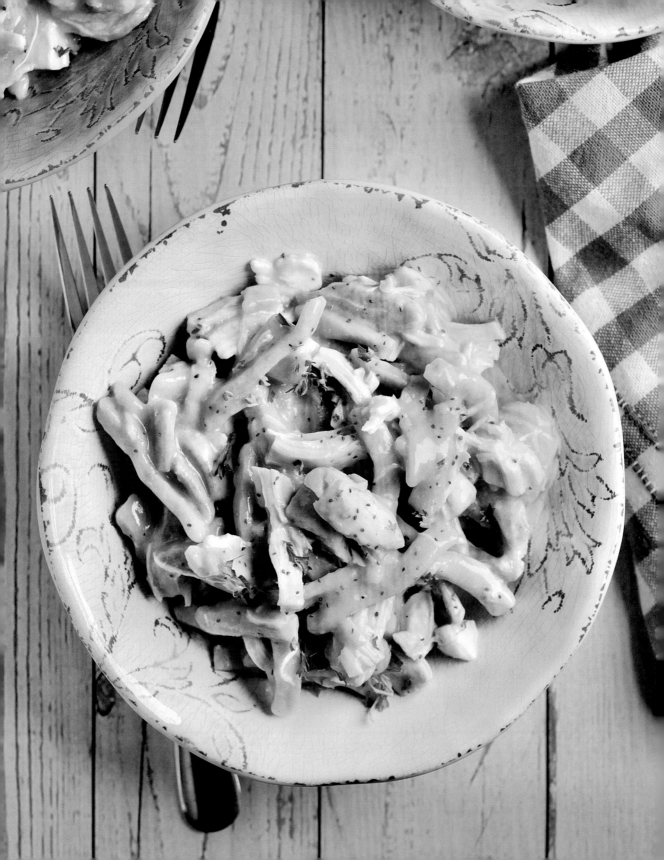

Chicken and Egg Noodle Dinner

Janie Steele, Moore, OK

Makes 5–7 servings

Prep. Time: 15 minutes ❧ Cooking Time: 6–7 hours ❧ Ideal slow-cooker size: 5-qt.

SLOW COOKER

1 lb. chicken breasts

1 can low-sodium cream of chicken soup

2 (15½-oz.) cans low-sodium chicken broth

1 tsp. garlic powder

1 tsp. onion powder

¼ tsp. celery seed

¼ tsp. pepper

4 Tbsp. (½ stick) butter or margarine

24-oz. bag frozen egg noodles

1. Place chicken in crock with all ingredients except the noodles.

2. Cover and cook for 5–6 hours on Low.

3. Remove chicken and shred. Return to slow cooker, then add frozen noodles and cook for an additional 40–60 minutes, or until noodles are tender.

INSTANT POT

Insta Pasta a la Maria

Maria Shevlin, Sicklerville, NJ

Makes 6–8 servings

Prep. Time: 10–15 minutes ⚬ *Cooking Time: 6 minutes*

32-oz. jar of your favorite spaghetti sauce, or 1 qt. of homemade

2 cups fresh chopped spinach

1 cup chopped mushrooms

½ precooked whole rotisserie chicken, shredded

1 tsp. salt

½ tsp. black pepper

½ tsp. dried basil

¼ tsp. red pepper flakes

1 tsp. parsley flakes

13¼-oz. box pasta, any shape or brand

3 cups water

1. Place the sauce in the bottom of the inner pot of the Instant Pot.

2. Add the spinach, then the mushrooms.

3. Add the chicken on top of the veggies and sauce.

4. Add the seasonings and give it a stir to mix.

5. Add the box of pasta.

6. Add the water.

7. Secure the lid and move vent to sealing. Set to Manual on high pressure for 6 minutes.

8. When cook time is up, release the pressure manually.

9. Remove the lid and stir to mix.

Spaghetti and Meatballs

Hope Comerford, Clinton Township, MI

Makes 6 servings

Prep. Time: 5 minutes   ❧   *Cooking Time: 10 minutes*

1 lb. frozen meatballs

8 oz. uncooked spaghetti

14½ oz. can diced tomatoes with basil, garlic, and oregano

3 cups water

24 oz. of your favorite pasta sauce

1. Pour the meatballs into the inner pot and spread around evenly.

2. Break the pasta in half and place over meatballs in a random pattern to help keep them from clumping all together.

3. Pour the diced tomatoes over the top of the pasta.

4. Pour in the water.

5. Pour in the pasta sauce evenly over the top. Make sure the pasta is completely submerged, pushing any under that may not yet be covered. DO NOT STIR.

6. Secure the lid and set the vent to sealing.

7. Manually set the cook time for 10 minutes on high pressure.

8. When cook time is up, manually release the pressure.

9. When the pin drops, remove the lid and stir.

Serving suggestion:
Serve with grated Parmesan cheese.

INSTANT POT

Beef in Noodles

Hope Comerford, Clinton Township, MI

Makes 4–6 servings

Prep. Time: 10 minutes ⚬ *Cooking Time: 38–40 minutes*

4 Tbsp. butter

1 ½ lb. stew beef

½ tsp. salt

¼ tsp. pepper

6 cups beef broth, *divided*

1 tsp. garlic powder

1 tsp. onion powder

1 Tbsp. Worcestershire sauce

1 tsp. low-sodium soy sauce

½ cup cornstarch

½ cup cold water

24 oz. egg noodles

1. Set the Instant Pot to the Sauté function and let it get hot.

2. Melt the butter, then immediately add the beef, season with the salt and pepper, and brown on all sides.

3. Add 1 cup of the broth and deglaze the pot, scraping up any stuck-on bits. Press Cancel.

4. Add the remaining broth, garlic powder, onion powder, Worcestershire sauce, and soy sauce.

5. Secure the lid and set the vent to sealing. Manually set the cook time for 28 minutes on high pressure.

6. When cook time is up, manually release the pressure.

7. When the pin drops, remove the lid. In a small bowl, mix the cornstarch and water, then add it into the pot, stirring.

8. Stir in the egg noodles and switch the Instant Pot to the Sauté function once again. Place the lid on the pot and allow the noodles to simmer for 6–8 minutes, or until tender.

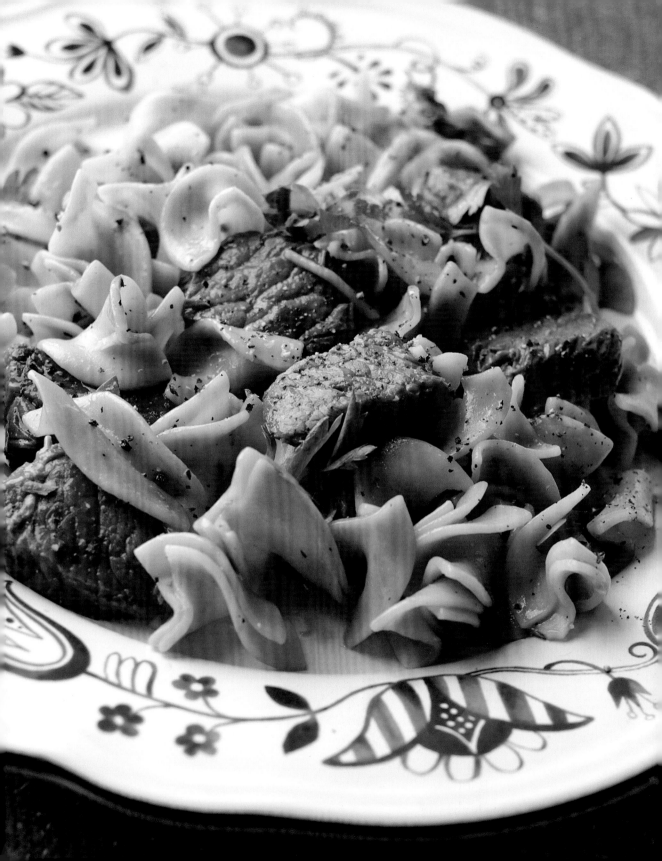

Fresh Veggie Lasagna

Deanne Gingrich, Lancaster, PA

Makes 4–6 servings

Prep. Time: 30 minutes ♣ *Cooking Time: 4 hours* ♣ *Ideal slow-cooker size: 4- or 5-qt.*

1½ cups shredded low-fat mozzarella cheese

½ cup low-fat ricotta cheese

⅓ cup grated Parmesan cheese

1 egg, lightly beaten

1 tsp. dried oregano

¼ tsp. garlic powder

3 cups marinara sauce, *divided*

1 medium zucchini, diced, *divided*

4 uncooked lasagna noodles

4 cups fresh baby spinach, *divided*

1 cup sliced fresh mushrooms, *divided*

1. Grease interior of slow-cooker crock.

2. In a bowl, mix the mozzarella, ricotta, and Parmesan cheeses, egg, oregano, and garlic powder. Set aside.

3. Spread ½ cup marinara sauce in crock.

4. Sprinkle with half the zucchini.

5. Spoon ⅓ of cheese mixture over zucchini.

6. Break 2 noodles into large pieces to cover cheese layer.

7. Spread ½ cup marinara over the noodles.

8. Top with half the spinach and then half the mushrooms.

9. Repeat layers, ending with cheese mixture, and then sauce. Press layers down firmly.

10. Cover and cook on Low for 4 hours, or until vegetables are as tender as you like them and noodles are fully cooked.

11. Let stand 15 minutes so lasagna can firm up before serving.

Baked Ziti

SLOW COOKER

Hope Comerford, Clinton Township, MI

Makes 8 servings

Prep. Time: 15 minutes ⚬ *Cooking Time: 4 hours* ⚬ *Ideal slow-cooker size: 5-qt.*

28-oz. can low-sodium crushed tomatoes

15-oz. can low-sodium tomato sauce

1½ tsp. Italian seasoning

1 tsp. garlic powder

1 tsp. onion powder

1 tsp. pepper

1 tsp. sea salt

1 lb. ziti or rigatoni pasta, uncooked, *divided*

1–2 cups low-fat shredded mozzarella cheese, *divided*

1. Spray crock with nonstick spray.

2. In a bowl, mix the crushed tomatoes, tomato sauce, Italian seasoning, garlic powder, onion powder, pepper, and salt.

3. In the bottom of the crock, pour ⅓ of the pasta sauce.

4. Add ½ of the pasta on top of the sauce.

5. Add another ⅓ of your pasta sauce.

6. Spread ½ of the mozzarella cheese on top of that.

7. Add the remaining pasta, the remaining sauce, and the remaining cheese on top of that.

8. Cover and cook on Low for 4 hours.

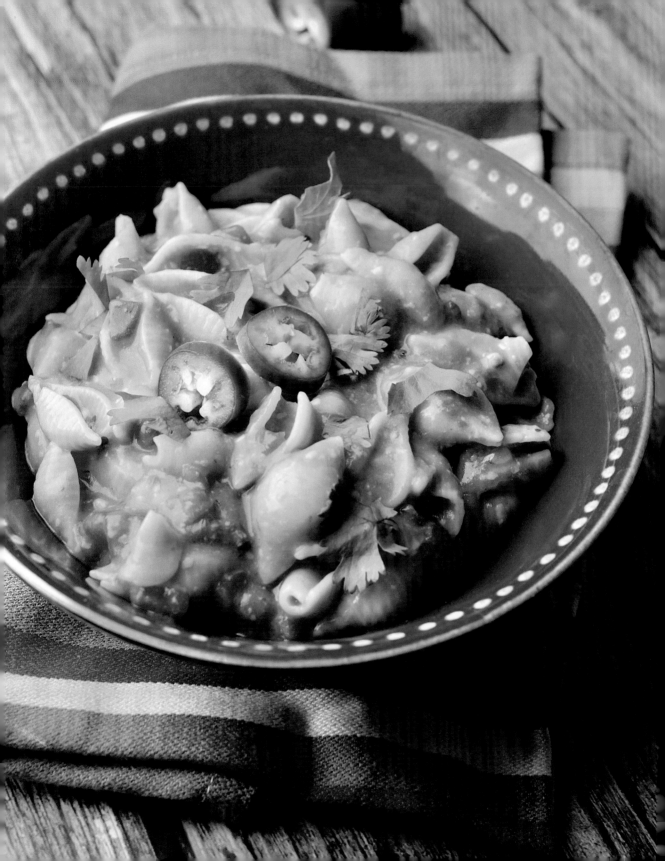

Creamy Mexican Pasta

Maria Shevlin, Sicklerville, NJ

Makes 4–5 servings

Prep. Time: 5 minutes ⚬ Cooking Time: 6 minutes

1 Tbsp. olive oil

½ sweet onion, diced

2 cloves garlic, minced

1 lb. uncooked pasta shells, small or medium-sized

1 Tbsp. taco seasoning

1 tsp. dried cilantro

4 oz. tomato sauce

1 cup mild salsa

1½ cups chicken stock

¼ cup heavy cream

4 oz. softened cream cheese

4 oz. cheddar cheese, shredded

1. Set the Instant Pot to the Sauté function and heat the olive oil.

2. Add the diced onion and garlic and cook for 2 minutes.

3. Press Cancel.

4. Add in the pasta.

5. Add the taco seasoning and cilantro, then tomato sauce, salsa, and stock. Stir well to mix.

6. Secure the lid and set the vent to sealing.

7. Manually set the cook time for 4 minutes on high pressure.

8. When cook time is up, manually release the pressure, then remove the lid when the pin drops.

9. Stir the pasta to ensure it is mixed well and coated evenly.

10. Add the heavy cream, cream cheese, and shredded cheese and stir until the cheese has melted.

Serving suggestion:
Top with sour cream and sliced scallions.

OVEN

Baked Macaroni

Ann Good, Perry, NY

Makes 12 servings

Prep. Time: 5 minutes   ⚘   *Baking Time: 3 hours*

6 Tbsp. (¾ stick) butter, melted

3 cups uncooked macaroni

2 qt. milk

4 cups shredded cheese of your choice

2 tsp. salt

½ tsp. pepper

1. In large bowl, mix the butter, macaroni, milk, cheese, salt, and pepper.

2. Pour the mixture into a greased 9 × 13-inch casserole dish.

3. Cover. Bake at 225°F for 2¾ hours.

4. Remove the cover. Bake for 15 minutes longer to brown the dish.

Tuna Noodle Casserole

Hope Comerford, Clinton Township, MI

Makes 8 servings

Prep. Time: 10 minutes & Cooking Time: 2 minutes

4 cups chicken broth

1 tsp. sea salt

1 tsp. garlic powder

1 tsp. onion powder

¼ tsp. pepper

12 oz. egg noodles

2 (5-oz.) cans tuna, drained

2 cups frozen peas and carrots, thawed

½ cup heavy cream

3 cups shredded white cheddar cheese

1. Pour the broth, salt, garlic powder, onion powder, and pepper into the inner pot of the Instant Pot. Stir.

2. Pour in the egg noodles and push under the liquid. Sprinkle the tuna on top.

3. Secure the lid and set the vent to sealing.

4. Manually set the cook time for 2 minutes on high pressure.

5. When cook time is up, let the pressure release naturally.

6. When the pin drops, remove the lid and stir in the peas and carrots.

7. SLOWLY stir in the heavy cream, a little at a time, so it does not curdle.

8. Stir in the shredded cheese, a little at a time. Press Cancel.

9. Let the mixture thicken with the lid off until desired thickness is reached. It will thicken as it cools.

Hot Tuna Macaroni Casserole

Dorothy VanDeest, Memphis, TN

Makes 6 servings

Prep. Time: 15 minutes ❧ Cooking Time: 2–6 hours ❧ Ideal slow-cooker size: 3-qt.

2 (6-oz.) cans tuna, water-packed, rinsed and drained

1½ cups cooked macaroni

½ cup finely chopped onions

¼ cup finely chopped green bell peppers

4-oz. can sliced mushrooms, drained

10-oz. pkg. frozen cauliflower, partially thawed

½ cup low-sodium, fat-free chicken broth

1. Combine all ingredients in slow cooker. Stir well.

2. Cover. Cook on Low for 4–6 hours or on High for 2–3 hours.

Variation:

You can use farfalle pasta in place of the macaroni.

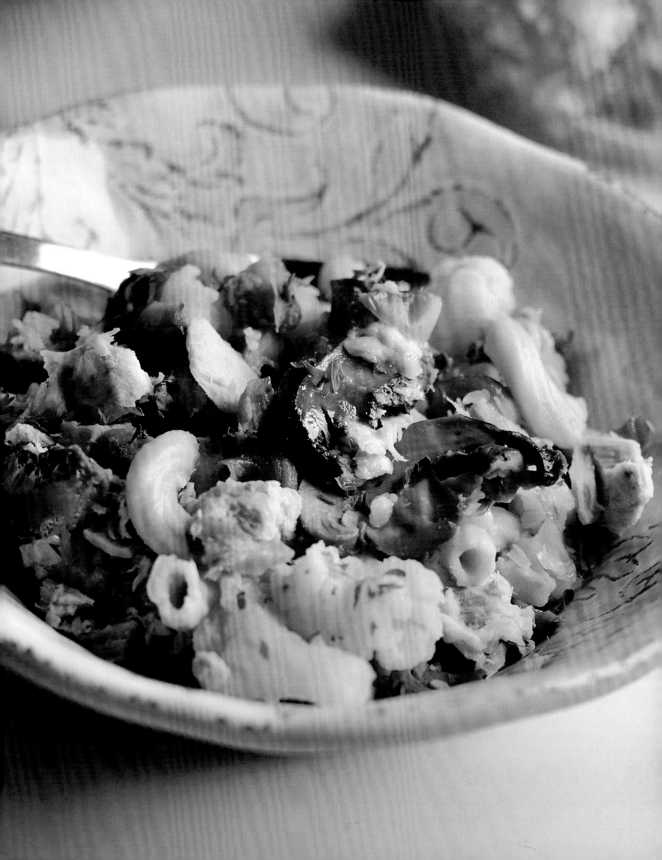

Salads

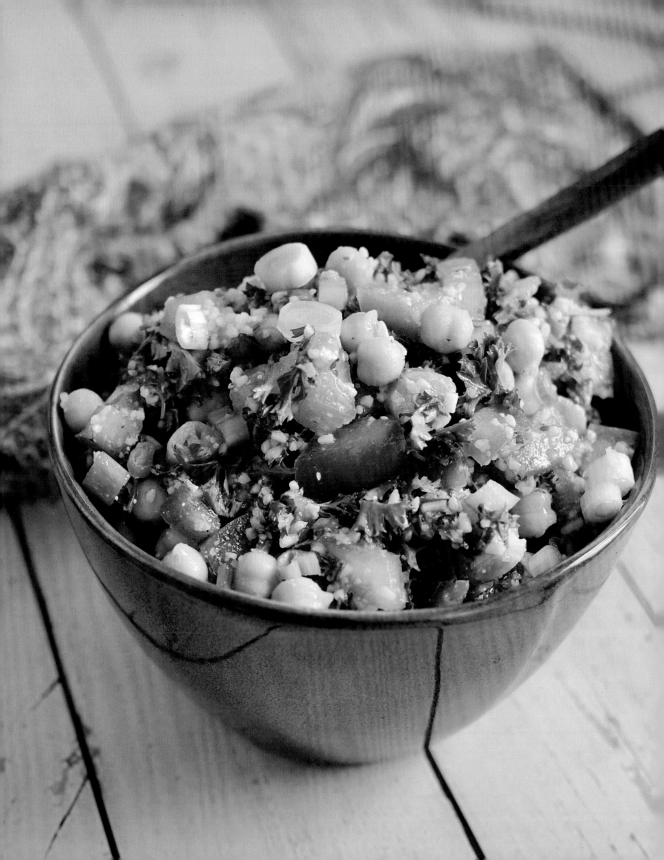

Tabouleh with Garbanzos

Jenelle Miller, Marion, SD

Makes 6 main-dish servings

Prep. Time: 20 minutes   ❧   Standing Time: 3 hours   ❧   Chilling Time: 1 hour or more

1¼ cups raw bulgur wheat,
or cracked wheat

4 cups boiling water

1 cup cooked garbanzos,
rinsed and drained

1¼ cups fresh minced parsley

¾ cup fresh minced mint

¾ cup minced scallions

3 tomatoes, chopped

¾ cup lemon juice

2 Tbsp. olive oil

2 Tbsp. water

1. Place raw bulgur into large stockpot. Pour 4 cups boiling water over bulgur. Let stand 3 hours.

2. Meanwhile, mince and chop other ingredients. Refrigerate until needed.

3. At the end of the 3 hours, drain bulgur well.

4. Add remaining ingredients to bulgur and stir well.

5. Chill at least 1 hour before serving.

STOVETOP

Lentil Salad

Sharon Brubaker, Myerstown, PA

Makes 8 servings

Prep. Time: 20 minutes ⚘ Cooking Time: 15–25 minutes ⚘ Chilling Time: 30 minutes

½ cup dried lentils

1½ cups water

15-oz. can garbanzo beans, rinsed and drained

4 scallions, chopped

1 green sweet bell pepper, julienned

1 red sweet bell pepper, julienned

1 yellow sweet bell pepper, julienned

Dressing:

1 Tbsp. lemon juice

⅓ cup olive oil

½ cup vinegar

⅓ cup sugar

1. Place lentils and water in saucepan and bring to boil. Reduce to simmer, cover, and cook 15–25 minutes, or until lentils are tender.

2. Drain lentils. Combine with remaining vegetables in a mixing bowl.

3. Mix dressing ingredients (lemon juice, olive oil, vinegar, and sugar) until thoroughly blended.

4. Stir dressing into vegetables.

5. Chill at least 30 minutes. Serve chilled.

Desserts

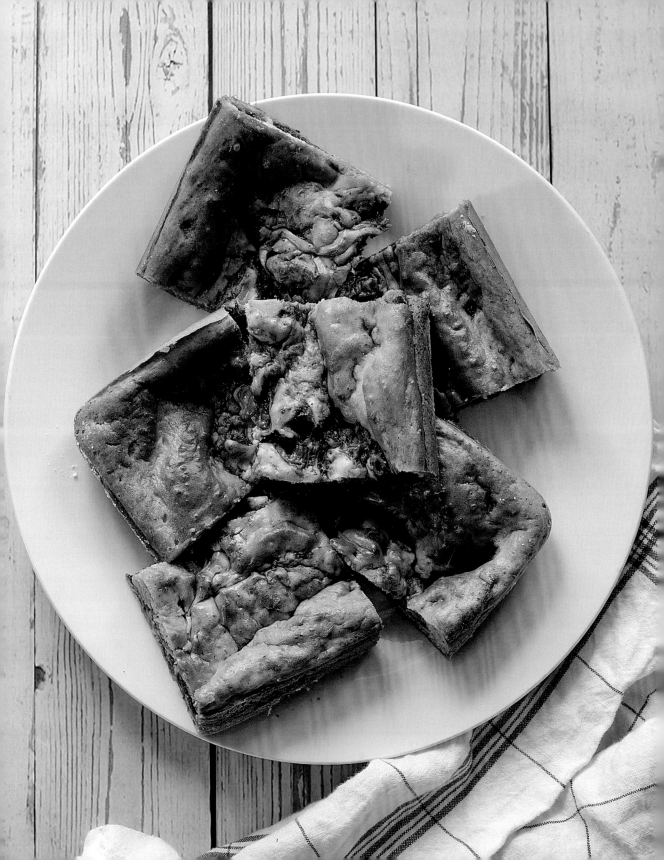

Blueberry Swirl Cake

Lori Lehman, Ephrata, PA

Makes 15 servings

Prep. Time: 15 minutes   Baking Time: 30–40 minutes

3-oz. pkg. cream cheese, softened
18¼-oz. box white cake mix
3 eggs
3 Tbsp. water
21-oz. can blueberry pie filling

1. Beat cream cheese in a large mixing bowl until soft and creamy.

2. Stir in dry cake mix, eggs, and water. Blend well with cream cheese.

3. Pour into a greased 9 × 13-inch baking pan.

4. Pour blueberry pie filling over top of batter.

5. Swirl blueberries and batter with a knife by zigzagging through batter.

6. Bake at 350°F for 30–40 minutes, or until tester inserted in center comes out clean.

Blueberry Bliss Dump Cake

Hope Comerford, Clinton Township, MI

Makes 8 servings

Prep. Time: 10 minutes ❧ Cooking Time: 5–6 hours ❧ Ideal slow-cooker size: 3-qt.

2 cups blueberries

2 Tbsp. orange zest

I Tbsp. fresh orange juice

½ cup turbinado sugar

¼ cup cornstarch

15-oz. box gluten-free yellow cake mix

¼ cup softened coconut oil

4 Tbsp. (½ stick) butter, cut into slices

1. Spray crock with nonstick spray or line with parchment paper.

2. Dump blueberries, orange zest, orange juice, turbinado sugar, and cornstarch into crock and mix.

3. Pour yellow cake mix over the top of the contents of the crock.

4. Place the coconut oil and slices of butter all over the top of the cake mix.

5. Cover and secure paper towel under the lid to absorb the moisture. Cook on Low for 5–6 hours.

Pineapple Upside-Down Cake

Vera M. Kuhns, Harrisonburg, VA

Makes 10 servings

Prep. Time: 20 minutes ⚮ Cooking Time: 4–5 hours ⚮ Ideal slow-cooker size: 4-qt.

½ cup melted butter, or margarine

1 cup brown sugar

20-oz. can pineapple slices, drained, reserving juice

6–8 maraschino cherries

1 box dry yellow cake mix

1. In a bowl, combine the butter and brown sugar. Spread over the bottom of a well-greased slow-cooker crock.

2. Add the pineapple slices and place cherries in the center of each one.

3. Prepare the cake according to package directions, using the reserved pineapple juice for part of the liquid. Spoon the cake batter into the cooker over the top of the fruit.

4. Cover the cooker with 2 tea towels and then with its own lid. Cook on High for 1 hour, and then on Low for 3–4 hours.

5. Allow the cake to cool for 10 minutes. Then run a knife around the edge and invert the cake onto a large platter.

SLOW COOKER

Dark Chocolate Lava Cake

Hope Comerford, Clinton Township, MI

Makes 8 servings

Prep. Time: 5–10 minutes 🍂 *Cook Time: 2–3 hours* 🍂 *Ideal slow-cooker size: 4-qt.*

5 eggs

1 cup dark cocoa powder

⅔ cup maple syrup

⅔ cup dark chocolate, chopped into very fine pieces or shaved

1. In a large mixing bowl, whisk the eggs and then slowly whisk in the cocoa powder, maple syrup, and dark chocolate.

2. Spray a slow-cooker crock with nonstick cooking spray.

3. Pour the egg/chocolate mixture into the crock.

4. Cover and cook on Low for 2–3 hours with some folded paper towel under the lid to collect condensation. It is done when the middle is set and bounces back up when touched.

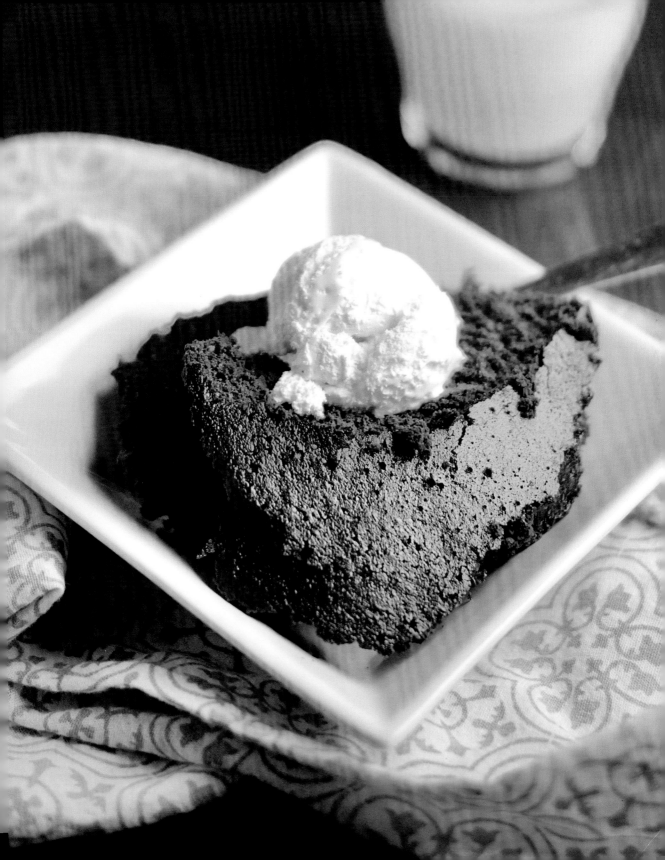

Peanut Butter and Hot Fudge Cake

Sara Wilson, Blairstown, MO

Makes 6 servings

Prep. Time: 10 minutes ⚹ *Cooking Time: 2–3 hours* ⚹ *Ideal slow-cooker size: 4-qt.*

½ cup flour

¾ cup sugar, *divided*

¾ tsp. baking powder

⅓ cup milk

1 Tbsp. oil

½ tsp. vanilla extract

¼ cup peanut butter

3 Tbsp. unsweetened cocoa powder

1 cup boiling water

1. Combine flour, ¼ cup sugar, and baking powder. Add milk, oil, and vanilla. Mix until smooth. Stir in peanut butter. Pour into slow cooker.

2. Mix together ½ cup sugar and cocoa powder. Gradually stir in boiling water. Pour mixture over batter in slow cooker. Do not stir.

3. Cover and cook on High 2–3 hours, or until toothpick inserted comes out clean.

Serving suggestion:

Serve warm and with vanilla ice cream.

Cherry Berry Cobbler

SLOW COOKER

Hope Comerford, Clinton Township, MI

Makes 6–8 servings

Prep. Time: 15–20 minutes ⁂ Cooking Time: 1½–3 hours ⁂ Ideal slow-cooker size: 3- to 5-qt.

8 Tbsp. (1 stick) butter, melted
1 cup flour
1 cup milk
1 cup turbinado sugar
2 tsp. baking powder
¼ tsp. salt
1 cup blackberries
1 cup blueberries
1 cup cherries, pitted

1. Spray crock with nonstick spray.

2. In a bowl, mix the butter, flour, milk, turbinado sugar, baking powder, and salt. Pour batter into crock.

3. Arrange the fruit on top of batter.

4. Cover and cook on High 1½–3 hours. It's finished when the middle is set and juice is bubbling at the edges.

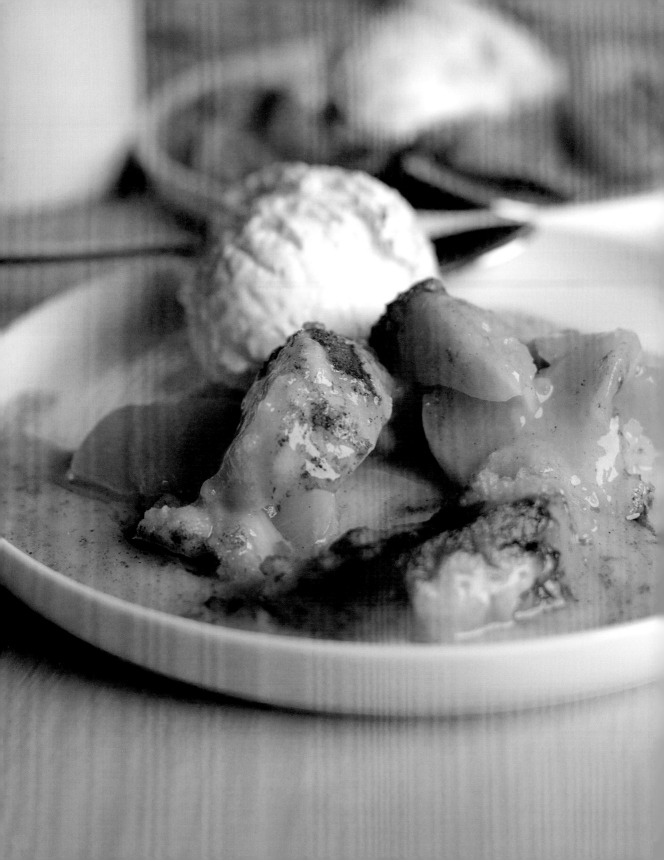

Peach Cobbler

Eileen Eash, Carlsbad, NM
June S. Groff, Denver, PA
Sharon Wantland, Menomonee Falls, WI

Makes 10 servings

Prep. Time: 30 minutes & Baking Time: 60–70 minutes

8 cups sliced fresh, or frozen, peaches

8 Tbsp. (1 stick) butter, softened

¾ cup sugar

1 cup flour

Cinnamon sugar (¼ tsp. cinnamon mixed with ½ tsp. sugar)

1. Place peaches in ungreased 9 × 13-inch baking dish.

2. In a medium-sized mixing bowl, cream butter and sugar together, either with a spoon or an electric mixer.

3. Add flour and mix well. Sprinkle over peaches.

4. Top with cinnamon sugar.

5. Bake at 325°F for 60–70 minutes, or until top is golden brown.

6. Serve warm with milk or ice cream, if you wish.

SLOW COOKER

Apple Crisp

Mary Jane Musser, Manheim, PA

Makes 6 servings

Prep. Time: 15–20 minutes ⚬ Cooking Time: 2–4 hours ⚬ Ideal slow-cooker size: 3-qt.

6 cups peeled, cored, and sliced cooking apples
½ cup dry quick oatmeal
½ cup brown sugar
½ cup flour
1 Tbsp. butter, softened
½ tsp. ground cinnamon

1. Place apples in slow cooker sprayed with nonfat cooking spray.

2. Combine remaining ingredients in mixing bowl until crumbly.

3. Sprinkle mixture over apples.

4. Cover. Cook on Low 4 hours or on High 2 hours.

Cherry Cheesecake Tarts

Jan Mast, Lancaster, PA

Makes 18 servings

Prep. Time: 15 minutes ⚬ Baking Time: 15–20 minutes

18 vanilla wafers

8 oz. cream cheese, softened

3 eggs

¾ cup sugar

21-oz. can cherry pie filling

Tips:

- Substitute blueberry pie filling or eliminate pie filling and use assorted fresh fruits, such as kiwi slices, orange slices, or strawberries.

- Refrigerate after preparing.

- Do not overbeat the cream cheese mixture—it needs to be heavy enough to keep the wafers at the bottom. If too much air is beaten into it, the wafers will float to the top.

1. Fill 18 cupcake tins with paper cupcake liners.

2. Place 1 vanilla wafer in each paper liner. Set aside.

3. Beat the cream cheese just until soft and smooth. Do not overbeat.

4. Add the eggs and sugar to the beaten cream cheese, beating until just blended. Do not overbeat.

5. Pour the cream cheese mixture evenly into 18 cupcake liners, covering the vanilla wafers.

6. Bake at 325°F for 15–20 minutes. Cool completely.

7. Top each cooled tart with cherry pie filling.

OVEN

Chocolate Chip Cheesecake

Chris Kaczynski, Schenectady, NY

Makes 16 servings

Prep. Time: 15 minutes & Baking Time: 45–50 minutes & Chilling Time: 3–4 hours

3 eggs, beaten

¾ cup sugar

3 (8-oz.) pkgs. cream cheese, softened

1 tsp. vanilla extract

24-oz. roll refrigerated chocolate
chip cookie dough

Tip:

If you wish, when serving,
top with whipped cream or
chocolate topping.

1. Preheat oven to 350°F.

2. Place all ingredients except cookie dough in large mixing bowl. With electric mixer, blend until creamy. Set aside.

3. Slice cookie dough into ¼-inch-thick slices. Set aside 9 slices.

4. Lay remaining slices in bottom of 9 × 13-inch baking pan. Pat the slices together to form a solid crust.

5. Spoon in cream cheese mixture. Spread out over cookie crust.

6. Arrange the reserved nine cookie slices on top of cream cheese mixture.

7. Bake at 350°F for 45–50 minutes. Allow to cool to room temperature.

8. Chill in refrigerator. When firm, cut into squares.

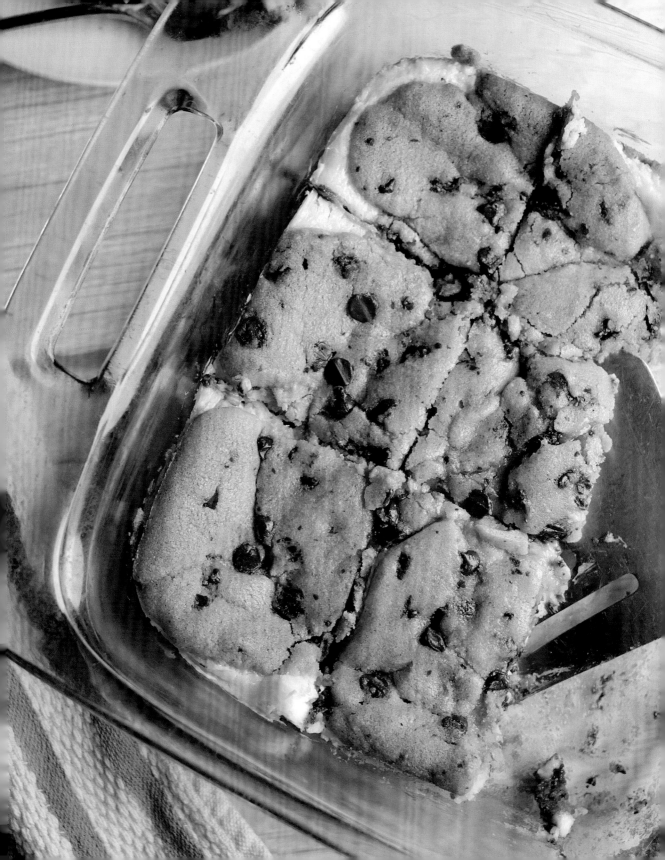

OVEN

Easy Brownies

Donna Klaassen, Whitewater, KS

Makes 36 brownies

Prep. Time: 15 minutes   *Baking Time: 25–30 minutes*

8 Tbsp. (1 stick) butter, softened

1 cup sugar

4 eggs

1 cup flour

1 can chocolate syrup

½ cup chopped walnuts, *optional*

1. In a medium mixing bowl, use an electric mixer to cream the butter and sugar together.

2. Add the eggs one at a time and beat after each addition.

3. Stir in the flour, blending well.

4. Stir in the chocolate syrup, blending well.

5. Stir in the walnuts, if using.

6. Pour into a lightly greased 9-inch square baking pan.

7. Bake at 350°F for 25–30 minutes.

8. When cooled, cut into squares with a plastic knife. (A plastic knife won't drag crumbs while cutting.)

Lemon Squares

OVEN

Mary Kathryn Yoder, Harrisonville, MO

Makes 15 servings

Prep. Time: 10 minutes   ❧   Baking Time: 30 minutes   ❧   Cooling Time: 1–2 hours

1 box angel food cake mix
21-oz. can lemon pie filling
⅛ cup confectioners' sugar

1. Mix cake mix and pie filling together with an electric mixer.

2. Pour into a lightly greased 9 × 13-inch baking pan.

3. Bake at 350°F for 30 minutes. Let cool.

4. Sprinkle confectioners' sugar over top.

5. Cut into bars.

 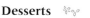

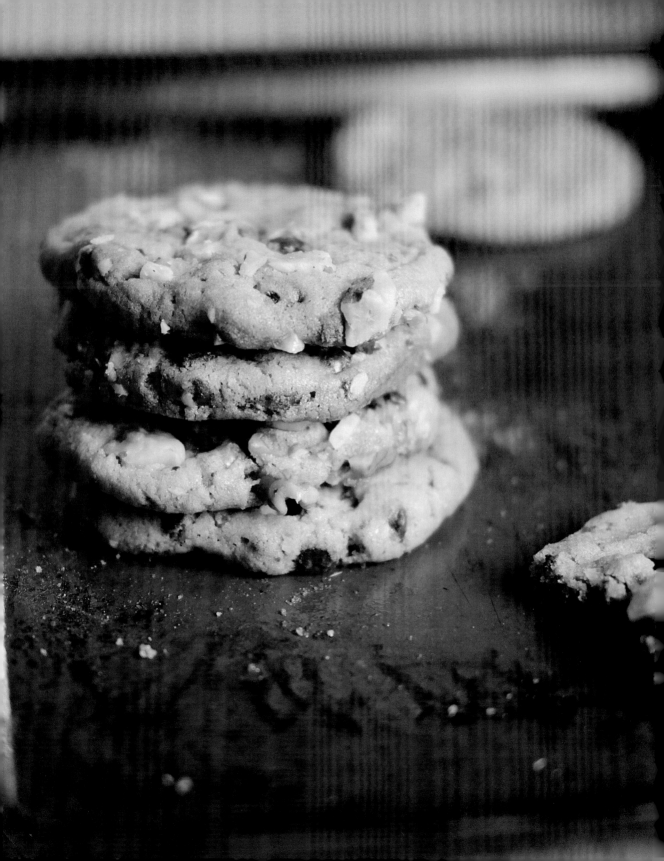

Chocolate Chip Cookies

Mary Martins, Fairbank, IA

Makes 3 dozen big cookies

Prep. Time: 15 minutes   Baking Time: 9 minutes per sheet   Chilling Time: 1 hour

16 Tbsp. (2 sticks) butter, at room temperature
1 cup brown sugar
1 cup sugar
3 eggs, beaten
3½ cups flour
2 tsp. cream of tartar
2 tsp. baking soda
½ tsp. salt
1 tsp. vanilla extract
12-oz. pkg. chocolate chips
1 cup chopped nuts, *optional*

1. In a large mixing bowl, combine butter, sugars, and eggs.

2. In a separate mixing bowl, sift together flour, cream of tartar, baking soda, and salt.

3. Add about one-third of the dry ingredients to the creamed mixture. Mix well. Add half of the remaining dry ingredients and mix well. Add the remaining dry ingredients and mix until thoroughly blended.

4. Stir in vanilla, chocolate chips, and nuts (if using). Chill in the fridge for 60 minutes.

5. Drop by spoonfuls onto a greased cookie sheet.

6. Bake at 400°F for about 9 minutes, or until lightly browned.

Tips:

- If you like smaller cookies, make the spoonfuls in Step 5 about the size of a level teaspoon.

- I usually bake a cookie sheet full and then cover the rest of the dough and keep it in the refrigerator for a day or so, so that I can have freshly baked cookies.

- Use macadamia nuts in Step 4 for a real treat.

OVEN

Peanut Butter Cookies

Juanita Lyndaker, Croghan, NY
Stacy Stoltzfus, Grantham, PA
Joleen Albrecht, Gladstone, MI
Doris Bachman, Putnam, IL

Makes 1–1½ dozen cookies

Prep. Time: 15 minutes ⚬ *Baking Time: 8–10 minutes per sheet*

I cup peanut butter
I cup sugar
I egg
Additional sugar

1. Mix the first three ingredients together in a medium-sized mixing bowl.

2. Break dough off with a teaspoon and shape into balls.

3. Roll each ball in granulated sugar.

4. Place on greased baking sheet. Press down with a fork, making a crisscross pattern.

5. Bake at 350°F for 8–10 minutes, or until golden brown.

Coconut Rice Pudding

Hope Comerford, Clinton Township, MI

Makes 6 servings

Prep. Time: 2 minutes   *Cooking Time: 10 minutes*

1 cup arborio rice, rinsed

1 cup unsweetened almond milk

14-oz. can light coconut milk

½ cup water

½ cup turbinado sugar, or sugar of your choice

1 stick cinnamon

¼ cup dried cranberries, *optional*

¼ cup unsweetened coconut flakes, *optional*

1. Place the rice into the inner pot of the Instant pot, along with all the remaining ingredients except the cranberries and coconut flakes.

2. Secure the lid and set the vent to sealing.

3. Using the Porridge setting, set the cook time for 10 minutes.

4. When the cooking time is over, let the pressure release naturally.

5. When the pin drops, remove the lid and remove cinnamon stick.

6. Stir and serve as is or sprinkle some cranberries and unsweetened coconut flakes on top of each serving. Enjoy!

NO BAKE

Snickers Apple Salad

Jennifer Archer, Kalona, IA

Makes 10–12 servings

Prep. Time: 15–20 minutes

3-oz. pkg. instant vanilla pudding

I cup milk

8-oz. container frozen whipped topping, thawed

6 apples, peeled or unpeeled, diced

6 Snickers bars, diced or broken

1. Mix pudding with milk in a large mixing bowl.

2. Fold in whipped topping.

3. Fold in chopped apples and Snickers.

4. Cover and refrigerate until ready to serve.

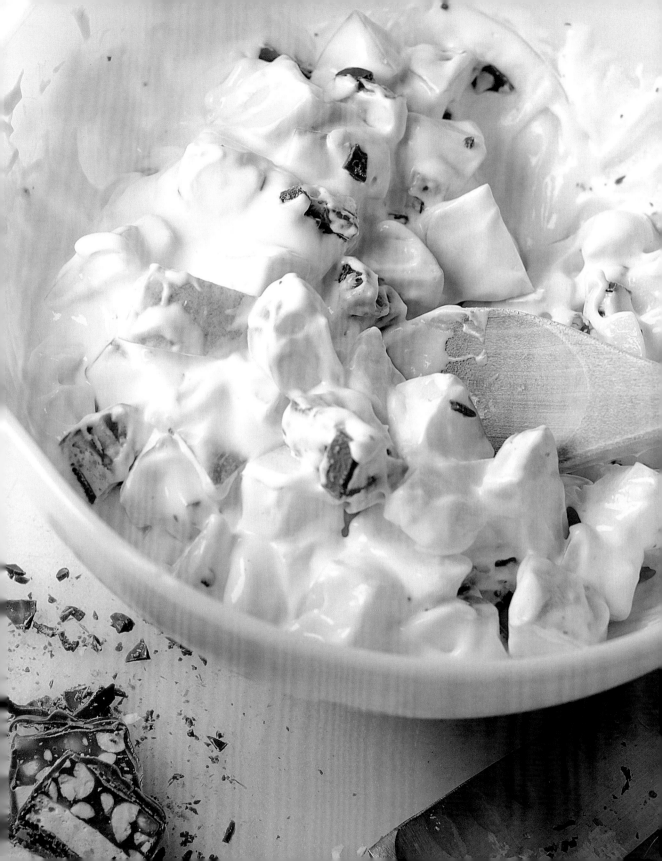

Metric Equivalent Measurements

If you're accustomed to using metric measurements, I don't want you to be inconvenienced by the imperial measurements I use in this book.

Use this handy chart, too, to figure out the size of the slow cooker you'll need for each recipe.

Weight (Dry Ingredients)

1 oz		30 g
4 oz	¼ lb	120 g
8 oz	½ lb	240 g
12 oz	¾ lb	360 g
16 oz	1 lb	480 g
32 oz	2 lb	960 g

Slow-Cooker Sizes

1-quart	0.96 l
2-quart	1.92 l
3-quart	2.88 l
4-quart	3.84 l
5-quart	4.80 l
6-quart	5.76 l
7-quart	6.72 l
8-quart	7.68 l

Volume (Liquid Ingredients)

½ tsp.		2 ml
1 tsp.		5 ml
1 Tbsp.	½ fl oz	15 ml
2 Tbsp.	1 fl oz	30 ml
¼ cup	2 fl oz	60 ml
⅓ cup	3 fl oz	80 ml
½ cup	4 fl oz	120 ml
⅔ cup	5 fl oz	160 ml
¾ cup	6 fl oz	180 ml
1 cup	8 fl oz	240 ml
1 pt	16 fl oz	480 ml
1 qt	32 fl oz	960 ml

Length

¼ in	6 mm
½ in	13 mm
¾ in	19 mm
1 in	25 mm
6 in	15 cm
12 in	30 cm

Recipe & Ingredient Index

About the Author

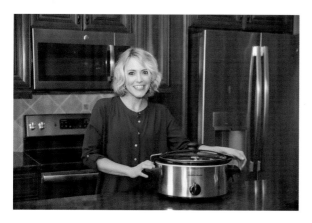

Hope Comerford is a mom, wife, elementary music teacher, blogger, recipe developer, public speaker, Young Living Essential Oils essential oil enthusiast/educator, and published author. In 2013, she was diagnosed with a severe gluten intolerance and since then has spent many hours creating easy, practical, and delicious gluten-free recipes that can be enjoyed by both those who are affected by gluten and those who are not.

Growing up, Hope spent many hours in the kitchen with her Meme (grandmother) and her love for cooking grew from there. While working on her master's degree when her daughter was young, Hope turned to her slow cookers for some salvation and sanity. It was from there she began truly experimenting with recipes and quickly learned she had the ability to get a little more creative in the kitchen and develop her own recipes.

In 2010, Hope started her blog, *A Busy Mom's Slow Cooker Adventures*, to simply share the recipes she was making with her family and friends. She never imagined people all over the world would begin visiting her page and sharing her recipes with others as well. In 2013, Hope self-published her first cookbook, *Slow Cooker Recipes 10 Ingredients or Less and Gluten-Free*, and then later wrote *The Gluten-Free Slow Cooker*.

Hope became the new brand ambassador and author of Fix-It and Forget-It in mid-2016. Since then, she has brought her excitement and creativeness to the Fix-It and Forget-It brand. Through Fix-It and Forget-It, she has written *Welcome Home 5-Ingredient Cookbook*, *Fix-It and Forget-It Healthy One-Pot Meals*, *Fix-It and Forget-It Everyday Instant Pot Favorites*, *Fix-It and Forget-It Weeknight Favorites*, and many more.

Hope lives in the city of Clinton Township, Michigan, near Metro Detroit. She has been happily married to her husband and best friend, Justin, since 2008. Together they have two children, Ella and Gavin, who are her motivation, inspiration, and heart. In her spare time, Hope enjoys traveling, singing, cooking, reading books, spending time with friends and family, and relaxing.